WHAT EVERY PATIENT SHOULD KNOW ABOUT HIS HEALTH AND HIS DOCTOR

Books by R. Douglas Collins, M.D.

What Every Patient Should Know
About His Health and His Doctor (1973)

Illustrated Diagnosis of Systemic Disease (1972)

Illustrated Manual of Laboratory Diagnosis (1968)

Illustrated Manual of Neurologic Diagnosis (1962)

WHAT EVERY PATIENT SHOULD KNOW ABOUT HIS HEALTH AND HIS DOCTOR

A GUIDE TO SYMPTOMS,
COMMON DISEASES, DIAGNOSTIC TESTS,
MEDICATIONS AND TREATMENTS,
HOME HEALTH CARE
AND THE PERIODS OF LIFE

R. DOUGLAS COLLINS, M.D.

AN EXPOSITION-BANNER BOOK
Exposition Press New York

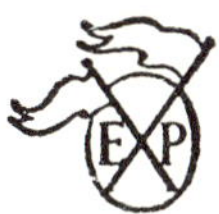

FIRST EDITION

Inquiries should be addressed to Exposition Press, Inc., 50 Jericho Turnpike, Jericho, N. Y. 11753

LIBRARY OF CONGRESS CATALOG CARD NUMBER: 73-82084

ISBN 0-682-47736-2

Manufactured in the United States of America
Published simultaneously in Canada by Transcanada Books

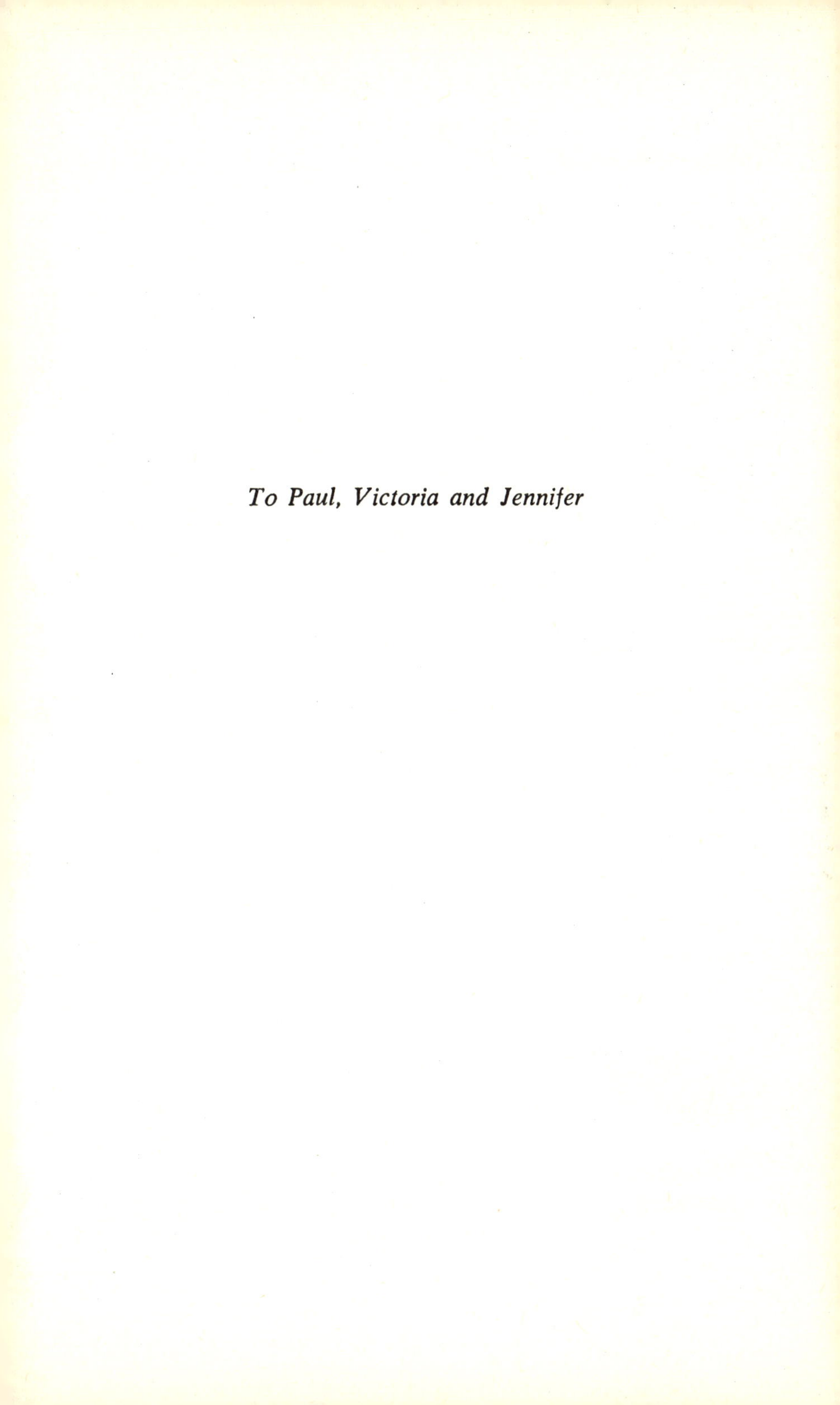

To Paul, Victoria and Jennifer

Contents

COMMON DISEASES

DIAGNOSTIC TESTS

MEDICATIONS AND TREATMENTS

HOME HEALTH CARE

PERIODS OF LIFE

Preface

Fifty years ago the old country doctor could walk into a home, look at the patient, give him a shot or a bag of pills and walk out without saying a word. Can anyone imagine this happening today?

Patients are no longer ignorant. They read about diseases in the newspapers and magazines. They watch television and movies about medicine and they want to know the facts. They want to know the cause of their illness, how to treat it, how to prevent it and what to expect in the future. They also want to know more about doctors, hospitals, nurses, and medical economics.

To date I have found no book that adequately answers these questions in an easy, understandable way. Thus, I must spend valuable time answering patients' questions myself.

This book is written to answer the most commonly asked questions about disease and medicine in general. For each disease the following six questions are asked and then answered in a simple, organized fashion.

1. What is it?
2. What causes it?
3. What are the symptoms and signs of it?
4. What can I do about it?
5. Is it dangerous?
6. What can I do to prevent it?

This is not a "do-it-yourself diagnosis and treatment" manual. Mainly it will help you help your physician get you well. By answering your questions it will allay fears, hopefully preventing new ones from developing in the process (in contrast to so many magazine and newspaper articles). The doctor-patient relationship can be strengthened by such understanding. Furthermore, prevention of illness may be best attacked in a book of this nature.

Of the many people who have assisted me in this manuscript I wish to thank especially Janice Dyer, R.N., and Dolly McAfee for typing the manuscript promptly and clearly.

R. DOUGLAS COLLINS, M.D.

THE DOCTOR'S WORLD

Doctors' Problems

Why don't doctors keep their appointments on schedule?

Many people can't understand why they must wait in the doctor's office. One simple reason is that in the average doctor's day at least two to three bona fide emergencies occur that he cannot anticipate or prevent. A patient may go into shock, a mother may go into labor, or emergency surgery must be performed. In addition to real emergencies, some unscheduled patients must be seen during scheduled office hours because their problems can't wait another day. For example, patients with fever, sore throat, diarrhea, etc., can't be told to wait. I may have as many as six to ten of these cases a day. We have to squeeze these patients in. This means patients being seen for routine follow-up care must wait. Occasionally hospital staff meetings must be scheduled in the middle of office hours, delaying our schedule.

However, a patient should not have to wait more than half an hour for a doctor. In my office we have a sign that says if you are waiting more than half an hour, please feel free to ask the receptionist for another appointment and leave. If the patient must see the doctor that day then I'm sure he won't mind waiting longer.

Not too many years ago doctors did not give appointments but simply took patients on a first-come, first-serve basis. Some doctors still do this. Under these circumstances a patient might wait as long as six hours for the doctor. At least the appointment system has improved this situation.

Why are doctor's fees so high?

A doctor's fees are high for six reasons: because his training is so long and expensive; because of his office overhead; because of his high rate of income tax; because he deals with human life; because he is in demand; and because of the long hours he must keep.

TRAINING

A doctor's training lasts from nine to fourteen years. This includes four years of college, four years of medical school, a year of internship, and three to five years of residency. During the eight years of college and medical school he gets no pay. He must in fact pay $3,000 to $5,000 a year for his training. If he were a $5.00-per-hour bricklayer and invested all of the $10,000 he could make every year for those eight years, he could have $150,000 to $200,000 in the bank at the end of these eight years and get a guaranteed income from the interest of $5,000 to $8,000 a year for the rest of his life.

In addition, if he specializes he must spend another three to five years of residency in a low-income bracket. Here again, if he were a bricklayer and invested all his money he could be assured of an additional $5,000 a year without working. The average laborer in this country earns $10,000 a year. Add $10,000 to $15,000 to this and you get the starting salary for most doctors entering practice today.

OFFICE OVERHEAD

For every dollar a doctor makes in his office fifty cents goes to overhead. There is office rent, electricity, heat, one to three nurses or assistants, accountant, legal fees, drugs, supplies, etc. The doctor cannot treat a patient out of his bag in his home anymore. He needs expensive equipment and a pleasant modern office to house the equipment. He can see more patients in less time with a building especially designed for him. Electrocardiograms, x-ray equipment, etc., all make diagnosis more certain. He must buy this equipment and the patients pay for it. I have over $60,000 worth of equipment in my office.

INCOME TAX

Because of the graduated income tax, a prosperous doctor pays the government twenty-five cents of every dollar he makes in his office or half his take-home pay. This is robbery but it's true. The average laborer does not pay the government such a big chunk so he can't understand it.

DEALING WITH HUMAN LIFE

No value can be placed on your life. Your life is like a rare diamond, and you wouldn't want just anyone to cut a rare diamond you owned; you would want an expert, therefore you must pay. A few years ago a New York judge wanted the top urologist in a New York medical school to remove his prostate. When he heard the fee was one thousand dollars he complained bitterly. The urologist replied, "My young associate, who is very good, will do it for three hundred and fifty dollars." The judge replied, "But I want you." Like your body, a good doctor is like a Stradivarius violin: you can't put a price on him.

DEMAND

The old law of supply and demand is in effect today. Fifty years ago when there were more doctors per patient, office fees were twenty-five cents. Now there is a definite shortage, partly because doctors won't work a hundred hours a week as they used to. Therefore, since the demand is high they can charge more.

HOURS

How many people like being called out in the middle of the night and want to work on Sunday? Other laborers get time-and-a-half and double time for overtime. The average doctor works seventy hours a week. He can't spend weekends with his family and many can't take much of a vacation. He is a slave to the telephone, which wakes him at all hours of the night and interrupts supper and vacations. Very few people realize what a dangerous weapon the telephone is in the wrong hands.

Despite the above factors, doctors' fees have only doubled in the past twenty years, while the price of most other items has tripled. The patients' ability to pay has doubled, too!

The Family Doctor

Fifty years ago almost all doctors were family doctors. These doctors were called by a different name, the general practitioner. They were "jacks of all trades." They delivered babies, prescribed drugs for medical illnesses, and performed the surgery when an organ went bad. They were the family counselor and psychotherapist. Today with the development of specialization this breed of doctor is fast disappearing. There are fewer than sixty thousand general practitioners of the three hundred thousand practicing physicians. Who will replace this physician? There are four possible ways the void can be filled.

The first way is with multispecialty clinics to provide each service that the family doctor used to perform, with the convenience of going to one place. However, a great disadvantage is that in many such clinics no one physician coordinates the team and correlates all the findings in each department. The medical team needs a quarterback. The patient needs someone who he feels really cares for him as a whole person. Any one of the different specialists in the clinic could serve this role, but probably the internist serves the role best for adults and the pediatrician for children.

A second possible way to fill the void is with solo practicing internists and pediatricians. They can treat all of the common medical illnesses, act as family counselor, and refer patients to the appropriate specialist for other problems.

A third method to fill the void is by simply training more "primary" or "family" physicians. The American Academy of Family Practice has already set up such training programs, and indeed there is an American Specialty Board of Family Practice. These physicians deliver babies, diagnose and treat medical illnesses in children and adults, and do minor surgery. Some even perform appendectomies.

The fourth method is a technique that many people use without knowing it. That is, to latch on to any kind of doctor—specialist or general practitioner—and let him be your advisor and consultant as to where to go for each illness. Some specialists don't like to be pestered for this service, but most of them are willing to provide it if they are already treating you for an illness that falls in their specialty.

All of these methods have their disadvantages, but I believe the best method is a multispecialty clinic with an internist or pediatrician coordinator for each patient. This allows for the highest quality of medical care with a personal touch.

Health Insurance

This subject has received wide attention today from the president, congressmen, the press, and many lay organizations. No one should be without the financial means to obtain good medical care at all times. Just how this could be provided is the question. Our country was founded on the principles of life, liberty, and the pursuit of happiness. All three of these cannot be obtained without help. But our country grew to its present greatness because of the free enterprise system. Total government control of medicine or any other business in our country would stifle initiative, remove free choice, and distort the doctor-patient relationship. Today our medical system is pluralistic and is multiphasic. That is, the delivery of health care is accomplished in many ways. It may be provided by a country doctor, by a private physician, by a multispecialty group of private physicians, or by a health maintenance organization, like the Kaiser Foundation. To insist on one system under government control would remove healthy competition, deny patients the right of choice of physicians, and injure the doctor-patient relationship. Any system to be successful must not destroy the present doctor-patient relationship. Contrary to popular belief, that relationship is not based alone on the doctor's unselfish desire to help his fellow man, but this is one major factor. That system is also based on a doctor's *selfish* desire to help his fellow man. The doctor takes an interest in his patient because it is his patient who pays his fee, and if he does not get the patient well, the patient may switch to another doctor. That relationship is also based on the patient's desire to cooperate with the doctor for fear that he may have to pay more medical fees with subsequent visits if he doesn't. A system that guarantees the doctor his fee or his salary and a permanent patient regardless of the quality of his care cannot help but fail. Similarly, a system that guarantees the patient a doctor and hospital services without costs will fail because the patient will not be motivated to cooperate. Also the patient may use the services under these circumstances whether he needs them or not.

Deficiencies of the Present System

BLUE SHIELD AND BLUE CROSS

This is a private insurance, which may be paid for by your employer or purchased by you individually. This program does not pay adequately for office or house calls. It does not provide for periodical physical examinations. Many diagnostic tests are paid for only when the patient is in the hospital; thus, patients are often hospitalized unnecessarily for diagnostic tests. It does not pay for nursing home care. The number of hospital days are limited.

MISCELLANEOUS INSURANCE PROGRAMS

Most of these are like Blue Shield and Blue Cross. They do not pay for office or house calls. They do not pay for periodic physical examinations, and they only provide diagnostic services when performed in the hospital. They also have a limited number of hospital days and do not pay for nursing home care.

MEDICARE

This plan has very few deficiencies. Medicare pays for office and house calls. It pays for outpatient diagnostic tests. It pays for periodic physicals. That is why, contrary to prediction by many experts, hospitals have not been overloaded since the plan came into effect. Unfortunately it is a government-controlled plan and it could be restricted should the government funds become limited. The number of hospital days are limited. Free choice of the physician is preserved.

Unfortunately, enrollment is limited to those people of sixty-five years of age or older with few exceptions.

MEDICAID

Enrollment in this program is limited to the poor. It is a government-controlled program subject to alterations according to budget and politics of the government. This program pays only one-half of the doctor's fees for office and house calls. It does not pay for all outpatient diagnostic tests unless performed in the outpatient department of a hospital. It pays for an unlimited number of days in a hospital. There is free choice of physicians, but some physicians refuse to take care of the patients under this program because the fees are too low.

CATASTROPHIC MEDICAL INSURANCE

This is available through many private insurance companies. It may be purchased by the individual or by a corporation in some cases. The program pays for all medical expenses over a deductible base of two hundred to five hundred dollars for any one illness, or in some cases for any one year, and pays up to as much as fifteen thousand dollars a year. After the deductible has been reached, house calls, office calls, diagnostic tests, surgical fees and hospitalization are all paid for.

KAISER FOUNDATION AND ALLIED PLANS

These are privately formed health maintenance organizations ("H.M.O."). Like Blue Shield and Blue Cross the plan is usually paid for by the employer, but it may be contracted by the individual privately. All medical expenses, office calls, diagnostic tests, surgical fees, and hospital services are paid for, but most of these organizations don't do house calls.

Nursing home care is not usually paid for. These organizations provide periodic physical examinations and vaccinations when indicated. Free choice of physician is denied in most cases because you must use the physician who is paid the salary by the organization.

WHAT PLAN SHOULD BE UNIVERSALLY APPLIED?

This may be a difficult question to answer. I personally believe everyone should have catastrophic medical insurance provided by a private insurance company and paid for partly by his employer and partly by the person himself, according to his ability to pay. The government may provide tax credits to the corporation or the individual to help defray these costs. Employers should also provide for Blue Shield and Blue Cross, but the program must include outpatient diagnostic services, whether they are in a physician's office or hospital, to avoid overloading hospitals with unnecessary patients. House calls and office calls should continue to be paid for by the patient. In this way he will not abuse these services and can maintain a free choice of his physician. Doctors, because of their unselfishness, will always adjust their fees according to the patient's income. Most doctors still scratch these fees completely when the patient demonstrates an inability to pay.

Free enterprise, the competitive spirit, and free choice of the physician must be preserved if we are to get the best medical care for the least amount of dollars.

Hospital

The hospital is a place for the sick, especially for those who are severely ill, to get intensive treatment that cannot be supplied on an outpatient basis or in the home. This intensive care may include frequent evaluations of the blood pressure, the pulse, and the electrocardiograph. It may include intravenous therapy. It may include major surgery, postoperative care of the surgical patient and delivery of babies, although these can be delivered at the home except in complicated cases. It includes hospitalization for frequent injections of antibiotics or other material that would require a nurse to visit the home around the clock if the patient were treated on an outpatient basis.

Today hospitals are also used for patients who require merely a diagnostic work-up. This may be justified if a minor surgical procedure, such as an arteriogram or a biopsy, is needed, since these people should have postoperative care. However, most hospitalized patients could have the diagnostic studies on an outpatient basis if it weren't for two things: one, that it is very convenient for the physician to have the patient in the hospital, and two, that the insurance companies are still oriented towards paying for diagnostic studies only when they are done in the hospital. This is absolutely absurd.

So today the hospital is not being used primarily for the severely ill. People do not go to the hospital to die, as they used to. Elderly or indigent patients are using the hospital as a custodial institution, where patients get a home and three meals a day until they are able to find a room in a nursing home. Actually, sixty to seventy percent of patients that are in most community hospitals do not need to be in the hospital at all. These are people who require only diagnostic studies, neurotics or malingerers, and the elderly, who, if they had proper facilities and had a proper home life, could be cared for at home. People who need custodial care could be cared for at home or in nursing homes, if there were enough available. Even some terminal cancer victims, who are kept on intravenous feeding for no more reason than to satisfy the whims of the family or the doctor's conscience that he is doing enough, could be discharged or nature allowed to take its course. In short, there is great over-utilization of hospitals today. This must be stopped if the medical care bill is going to be reduced.

Your Hospital Stay

Today your visit to the hospital should be a very pleasant one, particularly since most of the patients there are well enough to be ambulatory and are usually in a pleasant state of mind. As a rule, only in the intensive care unit are people found who are severely ill. If you are not going to the hospital in an emergency state, it is wise for you to pack your own pajamas, robe and slippers, and bring along a toothbrush, toothpaste, and cosmetics and other apparel that you desire to have with you. I oppose patients' bringing cigarettes or a bottle of booze with them, yet if this is the only way you can cut down on the anxiety of the stay, then I suppose it must be done. We do not like patients or visitors to smoke in the hospital. If you are coming to the hospital in an emergency state you often cannot bring your belongings with you, but you can send a relative, husband, wife or child home to pick these up to make your stay more comfortable. In most hospitals today a lot of these necessities of daily living are provided. Your meals are usually of superb quality and the beds are almost invariably comfortable. The wards of ten and twelve people are much less frequent in today's hospitals.

When you first come to the hospital you have to visit the admissions office, where you will be asked your address, date of birth, occupation, and your insurance coverage. Bring your insurance cards with you. Much of this information will be typed up on an Addressograph plate and sent back to the floor. You should show other means of paying your hospital bill today if you do not have Blue Shield or Blue Cross, or other insurance cards. Hospitals no longer specialize in charity cases, although it is true that occasionally a patient is admitted who does not have any money. There are funds in most hospitals that are provided for this sort of thing. After leaving the admissions office you are usually wheeled back to the room in a wheel chair. Sometimes you may walk if you are well and able. You'll often find your roommate very pleasant, as people are often in for a mild illness or diagnostic work-up. It is not likely that you will pick up any other disease while in the hospital, either, because most contagious patients are isolated in special areas of the hospital. Once brought to your room you should stay there. I dislike seeing patients walking up and down the hall or standing in the doorways looking out and watching the traffic. They are supposed to be there for a rest.

The first things on the agenda are *diagnostic studies.* The two most important groups of diagnostic studies are x-ray and laboratory. There will be a urine sample collected from you immediately by the nurse and sent for analysis. The laboratory technician will come early in the morning and draw blood, maybe three to four tubes. Most hospitals have rotuine blood work and routine urinalysis as part of their admission policy. A routine chest x-ray is often performed, but additional x-ray studies, such as an upper GI series (gastrointestinal), an intravenous pyelogram (x-ray of the kidneys), and a gall bladder x-ray are ordered at the discretion of the doctor. Your treatment usually consists of capsules or pills which will be given one to six times a day depending on how many times you need it. You may get injections. Occasionally you may get intravenous therapy. None of these injections or intravenous therapy are very painful and should be easy to tolerate.

Nurses

A very important element during your hospital stay is your communication with the nurse's aides and nurses. The nurses cannot visit you as often as they would like in today's hospitals because there are more demands from more patients. However, nurse's aides are always in and out of the rooms checking your temperature, blood pressure, pulse, urine output, stool, etc. By all means, do not hesitate to tell them any complaint that you have. When you have a complaint do not feel that you are a neurotic or something by mentioning it, because even though the nurse's aides may react with a little hostility, deep down inside they have a heart of gold. They understand that you deserve the best care, even though your complaint may sound very insignificant to them after all the patients they have taken care of during the day. If you are dissatisfied with the food or cannot sleep, please tell them! Also, if you are suffering from pain, please call them, and they will call your doctor and get something for the pain. You should not be uncomfortable in the hospital if it is at all possible. But your comfort depends on your speaking up. Many times patients wait till they see their doctor in the morning to mention these complaints. He is embarrassed and upset because they did not register the complaint early and do something about it.

Surgery

Before a surgical procedure, it is usually necessary to restrict your food after supper the night before and your drink after midnight. This is also true of a lot of the diagnostic tests and x-rays. The area to be operated on will be prepared with some sort of suitable soap, and it will be shaved. At times your privates must be shaved also, and while this is very embarrassing, it is the only way we can be sure the area is sterile. You will get a shot about an hour before surgery. This is usually a sedative to calm you down so that when you go to the operating room you won't be unnecessarily alarmed. Surgery today rarely lasts more than an hour or an hour and a half, and most procedures take a half hour to forty-five minutes. In the old days it used to take eight to nine hours to finish major abdominal surgery.

You will be brought to the operating room by a stretcher and transferred to the operating room table. Then the anesthesiologist may ask you a few questions about your history, put a blood pressure cuff on, and start an intravenous drip. He may then intubate you with an endotracheal tube, a catheter placed into your trachea. However, he won't do this until after you have been anesthetized and are almost or entirely asleep. We don't usually use anesthetics such as ether that cause serious postoperative symptoms, such as vomiting, etc. The newer anesthetics should make you very comfortable in the postoperative period. Before the operation you will be draped properly, so do not worry about your privacy at that time. More will be discussed about operative care in another section, but this is a brief summary.

When you are brought from the operating room you will be placed in a recovery room, and the vital signs such as blood pressure and pulse will be checked. Your intravenous will probably be discontinued before you leave the recovery room. When you first come out of the anesthesia you are usually dazed and sometimes get excitable and need to be restrained. This usually passes over very quickly, and then you start to feel very good and fall into a more natural sleep. An hour in the recovery room is usually sufficient to evaluate a patient for postoperative bleeding or other complications.

Then you are transferred back to your room. Here again you will be watched frequently by a nurse; sometimes the vital signs and urine output will be checked, but a lot of good postoperative care depends on you. If you do not tell the nurse that you have not moved your bowels for a couple of days, how can she tell the doctor and get the proper treatment? Do not think you are a narcotic addict just because you want your pain shot every four hours. Go ahead and ask for it! You won't be addicted that quickly to anything.

To the majority of patients the hospital stay will be a pleasant one, because you will be having diagnostic tests or oral therapy. Most patients do not require needles! When you are discharged you will probably walk out, unless you are in one of the hospitals that require you to be taken out by wheel chair, so that there is no liability involved if the patient trips.

In the hospital there are certain problems that we run into frequently regarding adequate patient care, and some of these I have already mentioned, but I would like to mention a few more. Some of the nursing staffs are smaller today, since there is a definite shortage of nurses. We hope that the patient can be a little more sympathetic towards the nurses. At the same time, do not keep your requests to yourself because there is a nursing shortage. Your needs are just as important, regardless of whether there is a nursing shortage or not.

The second thing that we have problems with are visitors. Visiting hours may run from two to eight o'clock or all day in some hospitals. Some hospitals restrict them to one to two hours a day. From the doctor's standpoint, the fewer hours of visiting the better. I recommend visiting hours be limited to one hour in the afternoon and one hour in the evening. Frequently I restrict the visitors to the immediate family, such as the wife, husband, or one of the children. I am against people trooping back and forth to the hospital to pay what is really just a respectful call rather than a call based on love of the individual. I abhor hospitals where there are visiting hours all day, or even for six hours. This is a detriment to the patient's health.

Another problem for the patient in most hospitals today is telephone calls. I feel that no patient should be called directly by phone. If the patient is not sick enough to have his phone calls restricted he shouldn't be in the hospital. The nurse may be called and the message relayed to the patient if it is important enough! There are exceptions to this, of course, i.e., a business executive who must keep in contact with his office. Usually this can be handled by his vice-president or some other associate. At times I have felt that it would be nice to have the phones taken out of the room and one phone placed in the hallway, where any patient who is ambulatory could make a call without disturbing other patients.

The fourth thing that seems to be a very definite problem in hospitals is the fact that the patient cannot get any rest because the nurses are running in and out asking questions (whether his bowels moved or whether he urinated) and taking his blood pressure. Early in the morning they may take the temperature and weight, waking him out of a deep sleep. Hospitals should have these things confined to a part of the day when the patient is least likely to be sleeping. There are many other things about hospitalization that I could discuss, but these are the major things that I want the patient to understand.

House Calls

Patients frequently complain or make humorous remarks about the fact that they cannot get a doctor to make a house call. Does this imply that the doctor is less interested in the patient's welfare today? Or are there other reasons for the disappearance of the house call?

From the patient's standpoint the house call is a very convenient thing, as long as the physician shows up when he is really needed. Many years ago the hospital facilities were inadequate, so the severely ill were taken care of in their homes, where they could be watched twenty-four hours a day by members of the family. They could be fed and cared for according to instructions that the physician left. Today the modern hospital has eliminated the need for caring for the severely ill at home. Thirty to forty years ago all of the medicines and all of the diagnostic equipment that were at a doctor's disposal could be carried in his bag. Today it is impossible to carry even all the medicines that are necessary for an emergency in a doctor's bag, let alone carry all the valuable diagnostic equipment along with him to the home. So any patient who insists on a house call when it would be more advantageous for the patient to be treated in the hospital or office is only cheating himself.

Form the physician's standpoint a house call is a very bad proposition. He must leave a busy office, jump in his car, drive ten minutes to one-half hour to the patient's home, sometimes spend fifteen to twenty minutes looking for the house number if it is dark, or try to read a map to find the patient's home, spend fifteen minutes to one-half hour at the patient's bedside comforting him, giving him the proper medication and treatment, and then spend maybe fifteen minutes to one-half hour with the family, discussing the condition and having a friendly cup of coffee. A house call can take anywhere from forty-five minutes to two hours if it is performed in this fashion. In that time the physician could see six to ten patients in his office, all of whom may feel that they need his services just as desperately. Even in true emergencies, when the patient is either unconscious or in shock, it is sometimes more advantageous to all concerned that the family call the ambulance and have the patient transported immediately to the hospital, where the doctor will meet him and administer emergency care. Ninety percent of those who ask for a house call, if spoken to kindly and considerately, can be convinced that it is better to be treated in the office or the hospital emergency room.

Are There Any Circumstances Left When a House Call is Absolutely the Only Way the Patient Can Be Treated?

Possibly a house call would be best for an elderly patient with a cold or sore throat, particularly one who has rheumatoid arthritis or some other crippling disease that makes it difficult to be placed in a car and brought to the office. Even this patient can be placed in an ambulance by experienced help and brought to the doctor's office or the emergency room at the hospital for their initial evaluation.

It is my opinion that patients and people in general should no longer insist that physicians make house calls.

The Ideal Doctor

Those of you who have watched *Marcus Welby, M.D.* on television have a pretty good idea in your mind of what the ideal doctor should be. Yet I think it should be laid down in writing as to what a physician might feel that an ideal doctor should be. I feel there are three important characteristics that all physicians agree an ideal doctor should have. These are availability, affability, and ability. Probably for the patient this is the proper order, too.

Availability

Fifty years ago the ideal physician was available twenty-four hours a day. This was his most important key to success and it was a thing that patients desired most of all. Patients desire this no less today. Fortunately they have other alternatives such as the hospital emergency room when they can't get their doctor! Or there are numerous other physicians that they can call until they find one who will be available to take care of them. Fifty years ago there was more competition. There were many more doctors per patient, and in order for the doctor to keep a patient he had to be available. On top of that doctors saw fewer patients per day fifty years ago. Therefore being available twenty-four hours a day did not mean that one was going to see that many more patients. Today physicians do not feel that they have to be available, since there are emergency room facilities where a doctor is on call twenty-four hours a day in most medium and large size cities. Also there is usually more than one doctor in most towns. Furthermore, they feel that many times when a patient calls them in the middle of the night it is unnecessary. If they were to keep themselves available for all these calls they would be awakened unnecessarily from their sleep. A study performed in London showed that at least sixty to seventy percent of house calls after midnight were unnecessary. Nevertheless most pediatricians, internists and family physicians today still maintain twenty-four hour telephone service and can be reached by phone as a rule. If not, they have substitutes in the form of a partner or associate who will take over the practice on those evenings or nights when they do not wish to be available. So I think today the ideal physician does not have to be available twenty-four hours a day himself, but he should make a service of either himself or an alternative physician available to the patient at all times, twenty-four hours a day. On the other side, the patient should realize that frequently his complaint can wait till the next day. If he wants to keep a good doctor he should be kind enough to consider beforehand whether his complaint is worthwhile calling the doctor out in the middle of the night. All physicians should have a twenty-four hour answering service. Any physician who doesn't deserves to lose patients in his practice. When on some rare occasion the associate or partner that the physician selects to cover him is not available, then there should be an emergency room physician available to the patient.

Reliability

Another important characteristic of an ideal physician that should be considered in association with availability is reliability. When a physician says that he is going to make a house call he should make it! Second, when he says he is going to be anywhere at a time to meet the patient he should get there without making the patient wait more than fifteen minutes at a time. There is nothing more frustrating to a patient than to have to wait an hour or two for a physician, even if it is not an emergency, when the doctor actually scheduled the patient for a certain time. This is true in his ordinary office calls too. He should never let the patient wait in the waiting room for more than a half hour without giving him the opportunity of cancelling the appointment and making a new one. There is very little excuse for a patient to have to wait more than a half hour in the average doctor's office today. If the patient is waiting longer than that, then the doctor is taking more patients than he should; or else he has been delayed unnecessarily in the day by errands for his wife, for himself, or by unnecessary conversation with other doctors and nurses at the hospital. On exceptions, of course, he may have a genuine emergency in the middle of the office hours, such as delivery of a baby or cardiac arrest, etc. But for a doctor to be chronically behind in his office schedule is uncalled for.

A doctor must also be reliable in calling patients back when they call the office for a discussion. It is true that most telephone calls to the office are not emergencies, but since the patient considers them important he should return the call within the same day. In my own practice I try to avoid this type of delay by taking the phone call immediately on anything the nurse cannot handle for the patient. This has been a big help to me, because at the end of office hours I no longer have a long list of patients to phone back. Another disadvantage in calling back later is that the patient may be out somewhere shopping or running errands and not be available. Patients today realize that a doctor should have time off to himself and to his family. They are not disturbed by the doctor's taking a vacation as long as he does not take more than two months a year, and they are not disturbed at his having weekends off as long as he provides coverage of comparable quality to himself.

Affability

A physician should be kind to his patients. The most important prescription that we have is kindness. It is harder for some physicians to show this than others, but a physician should practice being kind if it does not come natural for him. At times all of us, even those who have the warmest hearts, must make an effort to be kind, particularly to those patients who have chronic complaints, upon whom we have performed every conceivable study and come up with negative results and who continue to complain of pain or other aches. These patients are often referred to in our private conversations with other doctors as "crocks." Yet these people who come in with hypochondriacal and neurotic complaints probably need kindness more than anything else that we can prescribe. This kindness must be extended not only by the physician but by his office staff, also. The warmth that a doctor and his nurse provide the patient is really in many cases an excellent substitute for the warmth and kindness that the patient should have received from his mother or father, or perhaps currently the warmth and kindness they should be receiving from their husband, wife or their children. A little loving kindness goes a long way toward making the patient better, whether he is truly sick or whether he has an imaginary illness. Perhaps sixty to seventy percent of my patients who see me once or twice a month require love and kindness more than any of my other medicines. If the doctor is going to accept the responsibility of a patient's care, he should not reveal his hostility toward that patient when he discovers that the patient doesn't have a real illness or that he doesn't like something else about the patient. Every patient has something that is likeable about him. I find that I like many of them for their imperfections as much as I like them for their perfections. Occasionally anger does patients good, and therefore when a doctor feels angry with a patient he should consider whether it is valuable to express it. At times it may help that patient to lose weight or stop smoking or some other bad habit that they have, which will of course be very important to their health. If he is kind to this type of patient one hundred percent of the time then he will not be able to help them. Knowing when to get angry is a very important part of the art of medicine. A doctor who is available twenty-four hours a day but who shows up at a house call in a disgruntled mood is a detriment to his patient. It has been said that a bad temper is a luxury that no doctor can have, but a controlled temper is a very valuable asset. To be more specific about affability, I can describe how patients are treated in our office when they come for the first visit.

My nurse greets them at the door, asks them their name, gives them a warm hello, and tells them to take a seat and that the doctor will be with them very shortly. They are usually taken into one of the examining rooms, and a complete past history is taken on the patient by one of the nurses, who performs this in an extremely kind and considerate fashion. The patient is then introduced to me, and I always stand up and either shake his hand if it's a man or make some other form of greeting to show that we are interested in their problem. I do not like to open mail in front of new or old patients, and I do not ignore them when I come into my office, even though I may be on another errand. I do not like to take phone calls in front of new patients, but I do not mind handling a phone call in front of old patients, but I am very careful to keep the name of the patient on the phone confidential so that his privacy will not be violated. Our phone calls are conducted in an affable manner, also, even if they are two o'clock in the morning. One must be a very good listener with some of the older folks who have a difficult time telling something that might be very simple for someone else to describe. The ideal physician has patience, or he won't have any patients! The love that a physician has for his patients and the kindness that he gives to them can be seen very clearly by the attitude that his office staff has toward him. If he treats his office staff in the same manner then the air of kindness and love in the office permeates every nook and cranny.

The ideal physician must also be affable to his fellow physicians. This is more important for the specialist than for the family physician; but if the physician treats other members of the profession in an unkind manner, then it will soon get around that he is not a very likeable fellow. Patients will become suspicious of him, even his own. For this reason I do not talk down my fellow physicians in front of my patients. By blasting a fellow physician, I would be in a sense blasting the whole medical profession. A patient's cure is based just as much on faith in the entire profession as it is on faith in me, and I am going to disintegrate that faith by downing my colleagues in front of the patient. If I don't have a kind word to say about a colleague I refrain from saying anything to the patient about him. Affability is extremely important at the hospital medical staff meeting, where the diplomacy of kindness often gets things done much more quickly than adroitness or hostility.

A doctor often can demonstrate his kindness and love for mankind in general by participating in various service clubs in a community and also by his contributions to very worthy causes in his community. While the doctor should not demonstrate his generosity by blowing his trumpet, patients have a way of finding out whether he contributes very strongly to local organizations, and this implies whether he is interested or disinterested in their welfare, and in ways that might provide monetary gain for himself. On the other hand, it is hard to conceive that the ideal physician would want to run for public office, because then he could not devote adequate time to his medical profession, except in a few capacities such as school board director, etc.

Ability

The ideal physician should have an M.D. degree and an internship and a license to practice in his state. Most patients do not really comprehend what this all means. This has been shown time and time again, when imposters, particularly men who have a great deal of affability and a desire to be available, put up a fake M.D. license and start to practice medicine. These men build practices overnight, because they have the first two characteristics that I have mentioned. It is obvious that patients have very little means of deciding whether a doctor has ability or not. If he gets results, whether he is giving "sugar pills" or aspirin doesn't make any difference to the patient. This is probably why chiropractors still have a very good business. Their ability is not often questioned, and probably seventy to eighty percent of the conditions they treat would get better without any care at all. These men may have only two to three years of training, but patients don't ask questions about that. However, from his colleagues' point of view a physician must have ability. To get results in treating heart disease, diabetes, high blood pressure, tuberculosis, and other definitive diseases with definitive therapy it is obvious that a physician must have ability. If the physician cannot demonstrate ability to his colleagues, he will lose his hospital privileges and probably be removed from the county medical society as well. This will be sufficiently embarrassing to him to cause him emotional problems and further decrease his effectiveness as a physician. Patients can sometimes size up a doctor's ability by the way he handles them in his office and by his ability to answer their questions, but there are a lot of good "con artists" that without any medical training at all, except for articles in *The Reader's Digest,* are very capable of answering patients' questions to suit them. In fact, almost every patient or person has played the role of a doctor to his friend or acquaintance at one time or another by giving him advice, etc.

To repeat, the ideal doctor must have an M.D. degree from an established school. He must have an approved one-year internship; he should have at the very least a license in his state plus a membership in his county medical society and be on the staff of at least one qualified hospital. Beyond that, it is important to know whether he belongs to any specialty organizations. If he is a family physician he ought to have a membership in the American Academy of Family Practice. If he is a specialist it is important that he have evidence that he is board certified or at least board eligible (eligible to take the examination). It is true that there may be a few physicians that are board certified who do not have the affability or the desire to be available to make them good physicians. But at least we know that they have the ability to be a good physician if they have passed a special examination certifying them in their specialty. I am appalled at the number of patients who do not look for these credentials in the specialists they choose. There are some specialists who are not board eligible or board certified who might be very excellent in their area but you are taking a greater risk by going to someone who is not board eligible or certified.

A doctor's reputation in the community is often based on the number of people who claim that he saved their lives or cured them. Whether a patient is cured of a serious illness or not is difficult for the individual to prove without the assistance of other physicians who can look at the case objectively. A physician's ability can also be measured by whether he continues to write articles in journals, whether he has published a book, whether he attends meetings regularly each year, whether he is on the staff of a medical school, and the number of speaking engagements he is called upon to make. In the very near future it will be required of all physicians to take a recertifying examination or relicensing examination in their state, and this will prove the continuing quality of the physician. The ideal physician should be able to pass these tests with a breeze because he has kept up to date on all the medical knowledge in his particular area.

Confidentiality

A fourth important quality of the ideal physician is being able to keep matters discussed in his office confidential, and he must insist on this same confidentiality with his staff. If there is a security leak in his office, then he certainly cannot be classified as an ideal physician. At various parties or club meetings or even when entertaining guests in his own home, he will be asked about someone's illness or about why a certain patient came to him. He must quickly say that he cannot divulge such information but that they can ask the patient if they wish to. I refrain from divulging such information, even to close relatives, because many times the patients do not desire even their closest relatives to know. One of the few places in America today where a person can go and discuss his problems without having them spread all over the countryside is in a physician's office. The ideal physician should absolutely refuse to give confidential information to anyone without the permission of the patient. This extends even to testifying in court, unless he is given permission by the patient.

Other Characteristics

All of the other characteristics of an ideal physician can be grouped under one additional category, which I call creating a good image for the patient. A doctor's image to the patient would include the affability and the confidentiality and availability that I have already mentioned, but there are other things that are very important to provide a good image for a good doctor. First of all is his office! His office should be located in an attractive area of town that is easily accessible to patients. He should have plenty of parking. It is foolish, in my opinion, with today's transportation, for a doctor to locate his office near his home. For one thing, the patients may feel that the doctor's family, either his wife or other members of the family, may in some way find out about the nature of their visit or some other confidential information that they do not wish to have the doctor's family know. The office should be located in a modern building, or at least no more than twenty years or thirty years old. The interior of the office should be kept neat. The waiting room furniture, like all furniture in the office, should be up to date. The building should be soundproof. The examining room should also be soundproof so that there is no security leak. The examining rooms and consultation rooms should be large enough so that the patient does not feel cramped. The doctor's equipment should be up to date. This impresses a patient and often makes him get well just as much as the right medicine. A patient cannot have confidence in a doctor who uses shabby equipment or a doctor who has old broken-down chairs to sit in.

The doctor's office staff is very important to his image. They should be pleasant, courteous, trustworthy, honest, and loving individuals who have had paramedical training in whatever capacity they are serving him. If the aide does primarily nursing, she should have an R.N. If she does primarily laboratory work, then she should have laboratory training, etc. All of them should be neatly dressed. The doctor himself must be very neatly dressed, and I feel it is important during office hours to wear a shirt and a tie as well as a white laboratory coat or some other kind of white vesture.

The doctor should welcome patients with a nice greeting, and he should be courteous to them at all times. He should welcome all other members of the family to discuss the patient's problem with them. He should show patients their x-ray and laboratory reports and offer to give them copies of the reports and their x-rays at any time. I like to give my new patients a report of their initial findings and discuss all of their laboratory and x-ray results with them. I try to accommodate anyone calling in for an immediate appointment. We do not like to postpone them even if we do not feel it is an emergency. If a patient feels that he should see me a certain day I usually respond. I believe also that patients should be entitled to have consultations with another physician as often as they desire. This should not be an embarrassment to either the patient or the doctor. I offer to refer them to another physician for consultation even when I am certain that another physician cannot help them. I enlist the services of the clergymen to console patients spiritually when they need it. When I have to refer a patient to a specialist I always give the specialist a good build-up. This creates a good image of both myself and the referring doctor. The ideal physician should want to have all these characteristics. It is true that none of us fulfill all of these perfectly, but we should all strive for this perfection.

The Ideal Nurse

The ideal nurse should be at the very least graduated from an accredited school of nursing and licensed to practice in the state she is working in. Above all she should be dedicated to excellence in patient care and have a high degree of respect for doctors. Beyond this she should, like doctors, be clean, neat, intelligent, affable, energetic, resourceful, and able to keep things confidential. Finally, she must be available when needed. I cannot stress the importance of maintaining confidentiality enough. Today there is a tremendous security leak in our hospitals because nurses, orderlies, and nurse's aides are not instructed in this area.

Unlike doctors, nurses work only an eight-hour shift. Therefore there is very little excuse for laziness and a delayed response to the needs of her patients during her working hours. Unfortunately, nurses' days are so bogged down by paper work that they spend very little time in direct contact with the patient. Nurse's aides and practical nurses get much more contact with the patient. This is a deplorable situation! Fortunately, the innovation of ward secretaries has alleviated this situation somewhat. Other methods of eliminating paper work could be found.

There presently is an acute nursing shortage in our country. This has developed partly because of the closing of so many of the diploma schools. This is a real tragedy. Some schools are shortening their program to two years to meet the demands, but this is balanced by the fact that so many nurses are going on for their bachelors degree, which requires a four-year curriculum. On the other hand, practical nursing schools with one-year training have increased their number and enrollment, which has been a tremendous help. Like physicians, nurses now specialize, too. Thus there are nurse anesthetists, who administer general anesthesia during major and minor surgery. There are intensive care and coronary care nurses, who are especially trained to read electrocardiograms so that they can diagnose and treat acute irregularity of the heart beat under a doctor's supervision. Nurses can be taught to do many other routine tests that physicians perform. In fact, some doctors use nurses in their offices to diagnose and treat colds, sore throats, gastroenteritis, minor cuts, fractures, and other minor ailments. This saves them valuable time that can be used for attention to more severe illnesses.

For the above reasons I have the utmost respect for nurses. There is no limit to the many ways that they can help us.

Nursing Homes

Like hospitals of the 1800's and early 1900's most nursing homes used to be of poor quality. Today modern nursing homes are springing up everywhere. While Medicare has forced many nursing homes to improve their standards, all have not done so because they can survive without Medicare payments. More strict laws for state licensing are required.

For example, under present laws nursing homes do not need to have a house physician or even a medical consultant who makes regular daily rounds on the patients. Many nursing home patients don't see a doctor for months at a time. This is deplorable.

Nevertheless, many nursing homes have excellent standards, because their owners are either doctors or have high moral standards and want the best for their patients. The food, like that in almost any institution, often leaves something to be desired, but the rooms and beds are clean and comfortable. There are many other facilities to make your stay enjoyable. Some nursing homes are like a modern hotel, with the advantage of twenty-four hour nursing coverage. It should not be an insult to be placed in one of these.

We need more nursing homes badly. In my opinion, the government should have provided funds for both nursing home construction and financing a patient's stay long before Medicare was even conceived of. As it is, Medicare has failed to provide adequate funds for most patients and the limit of a hundred and eigthy days for each illness is a joke. Very few patients who require a nursing home ever get well enough to go back home. Providing food, shelter and medical care for the underprivileged elderly and anyone else who can't work and pay for it is clearly the responsibility of the state. Contrary to what politicians would have you believe, the American Medical Association (AMA) has never fought against this principle. Rather than spend their time pondering the question of national health insurance, the congressmen should be working toward this goal.

Many people experience a good bit of guilt upon placing their parents in a nursing home. This is uncalled for! There is nothing morally wrong with it. You may have an obligation to see that your parents get food, clothing, shelter, and medical care, but you should not have to provide this on their terms any more than they would let you do what you wanted when you were a child living under their roof. You should not feel obligated to keep sick or senile parents under your roof or in their own home under your supervision. If they resist going to the nursing home, constant efforts to persuade them by you and your doctor will usually be successful. If you can't allow yourself to put your parents in an institution even when your doctor believes it's best, then perhaps you need a psychiatrist.

Specialists

What are specialists?

A specialist is a physician who is fully licensed to practice all phases of medicine and surgery but in addition has taken three or more years of residency training to qualify him to specialize in a particular branch of medicine or surgery. Initially, there were men who limited their practice to either medicine or surgery. These were eventually called internists or general surgeons. Some who limited themselves to medicine went further and limited themselves to pediatric medicine. Today these are called pediatricians. Gradually internists, and later pediatricians, took additional training in a medical specialty, such as hematology (diagnosis and medical treatment of blood diseases), or cardiology (diagnosis and medical treatment of diseases of the heart), allergy, or the specialty of chest diseases. In university centers there are many more.

General surgeons began limiting themselves to surgery of a certain part of the body early in the game. Now we have eye surgeons (ophthalmologists), ear, nose and throat surgeons (otolaryngologists), chest surgeons (thoracic surgeons), brain surgeons (neurosurgeons), skin surgeons (dermatologists), kidney surgeons (urologists), womb and pelvic surgeons (gynecologists), bone surgeons (orthopedists), rectal surgeons (proctologists), and heart surgeons (cardiovascular surgeons). Undoubtedly there will be more. Many of these surgeons also treat diseases of their specialty medically. For instance, the ophthalmologist would not refer a patient with conjunctivitis (pink eye) to an internist. He would prescribe eye drops himself. This is all part of their specialty training in residency.

There are two specialties left that don't exactly qualify as a medical or surgical specialty. These are obstetrics (care and delivery of pregnant women) and, of course, psychiatry (the diagnosis and treatment of emotional or mental illness). The obstetrician is almost always a qualified gynecologist also.

Why are there so many specialists?

Simply because medical knowledge has mushroomed so greatly in the past fifty years that no one doctor can be proficient in all the treatment procedures in every illness. For example, in the 1920's we had no more than twenty useful drugs, and most diseases were treated with aspirin, sedatives or narcotics. Now we have thousands of useful drugs. Nevertheless, all physicians should be proficient in the *diagnosis* of any disease, regardless of what specialty it falls in. Unfortunately, some residency programs fail to emphasize this enough. That is why we must hesitate to shorten the four years of medical school. Just as important as diagnostic capability is the need for all physicians, specialist or not, to have a broad sympathetic understanding of his patient and life itself. We must be trained to care for the whole patient. We must be taught to be physicians first and specialists second.

How do I choose a specialist?

Many people are accustomed to asking a friend what doctor they should go to and who's the best. This may tell you who has the best personality or knows how to make money, but it doesn't give you his qualifications. Every year impostors are exposed, and recently some patients wanted one impostor to have the privilege to keep on practicing because he was so popular. The "yellow pages" can't tell you about a doctor's qualifications either. There is a directory of certified specialists, but only physicians can afford to buy one. The best way to select a specialist is to ask your family doctor. If you are not so fortunate as to have one of these rare commodities, then call your local county medical society for advice, or ask any other doctor you know well what you should do. Physicians rarely steer patients to a specialist because of a kickback. Their prime consideration is getting you well. It doesn't make sense to get a kickback of a few dollars along with a dead patient, when he probably could have made hundreds of dollars from caring for the patient over the years. When your doctor suggests a specialist ask him if the specialist is "board certified." This means the specialist has passed a thorough examination to be qualified in his specialty and is recognized fully by his peers. Probably less than two-thirds of all specialists have this qualification. Any doctor can call himself a specialist, but only board-certified specialists have proof that they are capable of practicing the specialty well.

Someday maybe the American Medical Association will publish a list of qualified physicians cheap enough for the public to buy. Until then the system I outlined above is safest.

SYMPTOMS

Blurred Vision

What is blurred vision?

By blurred vision is usually meant a smudging or clouding of the vision, but occasionally when a patient speaks of blurred vision he may mean dimming of the vision. It may mean blindness in some part of the visual field or double vision. Blurred vision is a very common thing.

What is the cause of blurred vision?

The causes of blurred vision are many. Probably the most frequent cause of blurred vision is a refractive error. In other words the lens of the eye does not focus properly to allow the image to come to rest sharply on the retina of the eye. This is the main reason that you see an ophthalmologist or optometrist. Refractive errors may be due to myopia, or nearsightedness; hyperopia, or farsightedness; presbyopia, a type of farsightedness that occurs in older people; or astigmatism, which is often hereditary. If the blurred vision is actually double vision it may be due to a muscle paralysis, either occurring at birth (called congenital strabismus), or occurring after birth due to a muscle or nerve paralysis.

There are many other causes of blurred vision that are not due to a refractive error. This is the reason that when a person first discovers he has blurred vision he should see an ophthalmologist rather than an optometrist. Only an ophthalmologist can evaluate you medically and also accurately interpret the diseases of the back of the eye through an ophthalmoscope.

Cataracts are a very common cause of blurred vision. Glaucoma, which is an increase in pressure in the eye, may cause blurred vision. Additional causes are diseases of the optic nerve or the retina. Brain tumors can cause increased pressure in the brain and swelling of the optic nerve. Certain systemic diseases (such as diabetes) may cause glaucoma. Diabetes may cause blurring just because of the increase in sugar in the blood. In addition, essential hypertension may cause blurring of the vision whether it be due to hemorrhages in the eye or swelling of the optic nerve. There are many other causes of blurred vision that we will not go into now because they are rather rare.

What are the symptoms and signs of blurred vision?

Of course blurred vision is a symptom itself, but usually associated with blurred vision there may be double vision, night blindness or pain in the eye. There may be rainbow rings around the eyes, severe headaches and many other symptoms.

What can I do about blurred vision?

The most important thing to do about blurred vision is to report it to your family doctor or ophthalmologist. He can evaluate you for a refractive error and decide whether the blurred vision is due to a local disease in the eye or to some medical illness such as diabetes or hypertension.

What will happen if I don't do anything about blurred vision?

Blurred vision if it persists more than two or three days rarely clears up without some sort of medical treatment or glasses.

Chest Pain

What is chest pain?

Most people who have chest pain think they have heart trouble. Some of my patients refer to left-sided chest pain as angina, but this should not be called angina unless it is definitely precipitated by exercises or confirmed by an electrocardiogram and other tests.

What causes chest pain?

Chest pain can be due to a variety of causes, as can almost any pain in the body. Most commonly chest pain is not due to any serious illness at all. It is often due to poor posture. It can be due to a spasm of the muscles in between the ribs, called "intercostal muscle spasm," or it can often be due to a mild inflammation of the muscles, joints, or ligaments in the chest wall. The more serious causes of chest pain are heart attacks (page 177), causing damage to the heart, or angina, which is due to a spasm of the coronary artery. Pleurisy is another serious cause that is due to an inflammation of the coverings of the lungs. Chest pain may also be caused by inflammation of the esophagus (the tube that leads from the mouth to the stomach). In this case it is often associated with heartburn, which will be discussed in another chapter.

Chest pain due to a heart attack is usually a pressure-like pain, radiating down one or both arms or up into the jaw, and is associated with a cold sweat and a feeling of impending death. This kind of chest pain is not increased by deep breathing, and there is usually no place one can put his fingers over the chest to create the pain. In other words there are no areas of tenderness over the chest.

A common type of chest pain that alarms a patient to thinking he has a heart attack is costochondritis. In this condition there are tender spots on the chest. In addition the pain is often increased by deep breathing. I can reassure patients over the phone when they call about chest pain that if the pain is increased by deep breathing it is not likely to be due to a heart attack. Sometimes chest pain is caused by arthritis in the neck or arthritis in the upper part of the spine. Another cause is shingles, which most people know is accompanied by a rash in the area where the pain is, although not always simultaneously.

What can I do about it?

Cases of mild chest pain associated with fever, generalized aches and pains, are usually due to a virus and nothing drastic needs to be done. When the pain is persistent, particularly when it is produced by exercises or associated with sweating, you should consult your doctor, who can establish a diagnosis of heart disease if this is the cause.

Is it dangerous?

It is dangerous not to consult your physician if you have a severe chest pain associated with sweating and radiating down your arms. However in ninety percent of the cases of chest pain the heart is not responsible and nothing will happen if you don't do anything about it.

Constipation

What is constipation?

To most Americans constipation is simply failure to have a bowel movement at least once a day. This is incorrect.

Three to four bowel movements a week may be normal as long as they are soft and do not cause any irritation of the rectum as they are passed. Constipation means the passage of excessively dry stool. A bowel movement every other day is plenty for the average American. We are used to one bowel movement a day because we eat so much more than we should. From infancy we are conditioned by our mothers that we should have a bowel movement a day. This leaves us with many neurotic overtones. Thus almost every American considers himself constipated if he does not have one bowel movement a day. Constipation is probably one of the commonest bowel complaints.

What causes constipation?

Constipation if it is on a pathological basis is often caused by spastic colitis. This is a condition wherein the bowel becomes very irritable and spastic, usually due to nervous tendencies. Constipation may also be due to cancer of the bowel and many other conditions.

The most common cause of constipation is psychological. The first time a person misses a bowel movement he begins taking a laxative and as he takes more and more laxatives his bowels become less and less responsive to them. Eventually if he does not have the laxative he does not move his bowels at all. Therefore he considers himself chronically constipated. A laxative habit is almost universally present among the elderly people in our society.

Constipation is sometimes caused by hemorrhoids or rectal fissures, because the person who has these conditions avoids moving his bowels to escape pain. Acute emotional shock can produce constipation because it inhibits the contractability of the bowel and slows the movement of fece, allowing it to have most of the water absorbed out of it while it is passing through the large intestine.

What can I do about constipation?

In most cases constipation will clear up by itself once the bowel regains its normal tone so that you can expel your feces. Of course if the stool is definitely hard and continues to be hard it is well to take something to soften it, such as roughage, mineral oil, or one of the drugs that your doctor can prescribe to soften stools. Keeping your bowels regular is an achievable goal if you take prune juice or other juices every day and/or drink at least eight glasses of fluid a day. A very good stimulant for the bowels in the early morning is one or two cups of coffee. This causes a gastrocolic reflex to go into action and the lower bowel is stimulated to expel the fece each morning. It the stool is very hard use a tap water enema. Suppositories such as glycerine or Ducolax may be used as well. High colonic enemas are to be discouraged. These clean out the entire large bowel and then the person does not move his bowels for another two days and feels that he is constipated when in reality he just has not had time to accumulate the fece in the rectum.

How can I prevent myself from getting constipated?

The best tip I give is to take laxatives only if your doctor has instructed you to do so. Also you should take more roughage in your diet, such as vegetables, prunes and juices, and drink eight glasses of fluid a day. A mineral oil or some other mild stool softener may be taken if you have been instructed to do so by your doctor.

Is constipation dangerous?

Constipation is not usually a dangerous condition. Once your body is able to establish normal reflexes and the bowels are able to move in a normal fashion, constipation will clear up. Occasionally constipation is due to intestinal obstruction either by a cancer, twisted bowel, or some other condition, but this is rare. In these instances you will not only not pass your stool but you won't be able to pass gas either.

Convulsions

What are convulsions?

Convulsions are spasmodic movements of the body usually associated with unconsciousness, lasting between one minute to a half hour as a rule, and often associated with frothing at the mouth, cyanosis (a bluish coloring on face and at extremities), and wetting of the pants. Of course some convulsions may be hysterical (a subconscious mimicking of a seizure by the patient).

What causes convulsions?

Convulsions are most commonly caused by idiopathic epilepsy, which is often due to a genetically transmitted abnormality of a few brain cells. It takes only two or three of the brain cells out of the eight billion or so that we have to produce an attack of epilepsy. Not all epileptic attacks are convulsions. Some take the form of just ordinary fainting. Some occur with just a sudden pain, tingling, or paralysis in some part of the body rather than an actual all-out convulsive movement of the whole body. But there are many other causes of convulsions. Brain concussion, meningitis, encephalitis, strokes and other types of impaired circulation in the brain may cause a convulsion. Convulsions may occur in diabetics either when they take too much insulin or when they go into a diabetic coma from too little insulin. Metabolic diseases of the kidneys and the lungs may cause convulsions. But, to reiterate, the commonest cause is genetic epilepsy. Of course the epilepsy can also be due to birth trauma or birth anoxia (shortage of oxygen) as occurs in premature infants or breech deliveries. It should be pointed out that just because a person is born with epilepsy doesn't mean he is going to have a lower than average intelligence. Most epileptics have average or better than average intelligence.

What are the symptoms and signs of convulsions?

A convulsion may be a movement of the entire body, usually beginning with rigidity, and then followed by clonic (spasmodic) movements of the hands, arms, and legs; or it may affect just one part of the body such as one arm or the left side of the face. It is usually associated with frothing at the mouth, biting the tongue, wetting of the pants, falling to the floor and unconsciousness. The patient usually does not recall the convulsion at all. In some cases when there is psychomotor epilepsy the patient may bang the table or scream or go into an hysterical state, but this is unusual.

What can I do about convulsions?

The most important thing is to see your family doctor and get a complete neurological examination. Often he will refer you to a neurological specialist for this, and then an EEG, a skull x-ray and a spinal tap are often performed, particularly if the patient is an adult, to exclude a brain tumor. If these tests are perfectly normal he will probably put you on something such as Dilantin, phenobarbital, or Mysoline. If the tests give any indication that you may have a brain tumor or some other disease of the brain, then you might require arteriography, pneumoencephalography, (in which air is injected into the ventricles of the brain) or a brain scan to rule out the possibility of a brain tumor or some other disease.

Are convulsions dangerous?

During a convulsion it is rare for a patient to die or to experience any permanent paralysis in his body. However, convulsions are dangerous because they may occur when you are crossing the road or while you are driving a car and thus cause accidents.

What will happen if I don't do anything about them?

If you don't do anything about convulsions you may not have another one for three to six months, ten years, or even the rest of your life, but in most cases without treatment you will continue to have them once a month or more.

How can I prevent myself from getting them?

Once it is established that you have epilepsy the best way to prevent it is by taking the medication the doctor prescribes regularly. There are other general measures you can practice. You should not drink too much coffee or smoke too much, and you should get adequate sleep. You should not hyperventilate when you exercise. In some cases your doctor will prescribe a diet that is high in fat. Some cases of convulsions are actually produced by unusual music or flashes of light, and therefore you must avoid these stimuli if your convulsions are that type. Of course, if the convulsion is due to a brain tumor, a depressed skull fracture, or some other disease of the nervous system then appropriate treatment must be undertaken to relieve them.

Depression

What is depression?

Depression is a normal psychological feeling in response to certain upsets in our lives. All of us have experienced depression when we break up with a loved one, when a loved one is transferred overseas, or perhaps when we have had to leave home for college. Men have experienced depression as a result of the failure of a business deal. These short periods of depression are normal and should not be construed as requiring intensive medical care. Women often express severe grief at the death of their husband, mother, or father, but men are more frequently prone to suppress this grief. Sometimes this suppression may cause a more prolonged and lasting depression.

Depression is one of the most common symptoms that I see in my office from day to day. By this I mean a type of depression that lasts for more than two to three weeks and begins to interfere with a patient's ability to adapt to his life. About one in ten people will experience this type of depression during their lifetime. This is three times more common in women than it is in men. Of course women, because of some physiological mechanism in their body, become depressed just before or during their menstrual period. This is normal and husbands should realize that a woman is going to be more irritable during this time and not be too sensitive about it. They must grin and bear the brunt of the hostility that is expressed during this time.

What is the cause of depression?

There are three types of depression that we consider medical problems. One is a "neurotic depressive reaction," which is usually a response to something that happens in the environment, such as a failure in business, financial worries, marital discord, bad health, the death of a loved one, or other personal tragedy.

Another type of depression, however, results from physiological changes in the body and is usually termed an "endogenous depression." These physiological changes are still not well understood. Some of them may be due to endocrinological changes such as the change of life in women. Whether the lowering of estrogen or other hormones produced by the ovary is the direct cause of the depression experienced during menopause is not definitely ascertained; but because of the excellent results of treatment with estrogen in women of menopausal age who have depression I would feel that the endocrinological (glandular) role is a big one. I have seen women who ascribed their depression to something in their environment, such as marital discord or loss of a loved one, improve remarkably on estrogen treatment. This indicates that environmental factors are probably not as commonly a cause of prolonged depression as we thought.

The third type of depression is labeled by psychiatrists the "manic-depressive psychosis." This type of depression is not necessarily associated with any endocrinological or physiological change but usually occurs in people who have an hereditary predisposition to this type of depression. In other words, their parents or someone in their ancestry have experienced a similar type of depression. These people also may have periods of elation, called a manic phase, in which they experience a flight of ideas, involve themselves in many different projects and are constantly on the move. This phase is often followed by an "exhausted" phase in which they experience depression.

What are the symptoms and signs of depression?

The signs of depression are pretty familiar to everyone. They usually include an empty feeling inside, crying or the desire to cry and may be accompanied by a loss of appetite and insomnia. The patient may report to the doctor that he or she has lost weight and just has no desire to do anything in life. Many of these patients have suicidal ruminations and some of them actually carry out the desire. There is often loss of sexual desire, but while this is usually an effect of depression it may be a cause of depression. Patients who are depressed complain more and more of various symptoms in their body such as stomach pain, fatigue, headaches, etc. Almost any "physical" symptom can be the result of a depression. Women who are depressed during menopause complain of hot flushes.

What can I do about depression?

As soon as a patient experiences any of the symptoms mentioned above, such as fatigue, multiple symptoms in each organ, tearfulness, loss of appetite or insomnia, he should report to his family doctor. The doctor can help depressed patients immensely today with the modern treatment available. In former times shock therapy was one of the few things that could be done for the depressed patient outside of permanent hospitalization. Now your physician has many, many drugs that he can use for depression. If your depression is due to some environmental problem he will be able to talk this out with you and possibly help you make some environmental changes to your benefit. This is not always possible but it is certainly one method of treating depression. If your physician feels psychotherapy will help, don't resist it! It doesn't mean you're "crazy," because most normal people could benefit from psychotherapy if they would have it.

More often, your doctor will prescribe a tranquilizer or antidepressant drug. We have several new and useful antidepressant drugs on the market. In women of menopausal age it is very important to prescribe estrogen hormones if they have a normal pelvic examination. It is often possible to estimate the amount of estrogen needed by a "pap" smear. There is also a urine test that can be done to determine the amount of estrogen needed. Often rest alone in a community hospital is of significant value in the treatment of depression. Simply changing one's environment can be of help, although doctors do not prescribe a vacation as frequently as they used to. Depressed patients should not be allowed to vegetate at home and keep to themselves. Some effort should be made to bring them into the family situation. However I do not advise this to be done to an extreme.

Is depression dangerous?

It certainly is if it is left untreated! As I said before one of the main symptoms of depression is suicidal ideas. These people don't just think about suicide, they try it! Many cases of depression will clear up without a doctor's care but it certainly is better to have a doctor's supervision while one is going through a state such as this.

What will happen if I don't do anything about it?

You will probably get over it in three to six months. Treatment will get you over it faster and help you avoid hospitalization, loss of your job and suicide.

Diarrhea

What is diarrhea?

Diarrhea is the frequent passage of loose stools. More than two bowel movements a day would be considered frequent; but since many people have three bowel movements a day, if the stool is not loose this condition is perfectly normal for these people. Diarrhea fluid may be green or yellow or brown depending on how active the bowels are. The more active the bowels and the more frequent the stools the more likely the color is to become yellow or green. Occasionally the diarrhea is associated with blood or mucus.

What causes diarrhea?

Diarrhea may be acute or chronic. The most common cause of acute diarrhea is a viral infection. This diarrhea usually lasts from twenty-four to forty-eight hours and is done with. However, foods that are allowed to sit overnight, particularly dairy products that are allowed to sit outside the refrigerator, may be responsible for an acute diarrhea due to staphylococcus poisoning. The staphylococcus bacteria releases a powerful toxin which stimulates the bowel to move frequently. Other causes of acute diarrhea are the relatives of the typhoid family, that is Salmonella or Shigella bacteria. These are uncommon in most areas of the United States because we have good clean drinking water and food. However, when you travel to foreign countries you may be more subject to these latter types of diarrhea.

The most common cause of chronic diarrhea is irritable bowel or irritable colon. In these cases the diarrhea alternates with constipation and there is frequently mucus in the stool and also severe intestinal cramps. This type of diarrhea is usually related to emotions.

Other causes of chronic diarrhea are: bad dietary habits; malabsorption syndrome, in which because of some disease the bowel cannot absorb the food; occasionally, cancer of the large bowel; hyperactive thyroid; Addison's disease; and some other generalized diseases such as diabetes mellitus. Ulcerative colitis (page 128) is another cause of diarrhea but in this condition it is usually associated with blood or mucus.

What can I do about it?

With acute diarrhea it is often unnecessary to contact your doctor unless you develop a fever. Without fever, the cause is usually a viral gastroenteritis and the diarrhea will clear up in twenty-four to forty-eight hours; however, if you develop chills or fever then you must contact your doctor because he may want to prescribe an antibiotic and take a culture of your stool. General measures for diarrhea are applying heat to the abdomen, restricting food intake to just fluid, and taking Kaopectate and possibly paregoric. Your doctor may prescribe something a little stronger such as Lomotil or another narcotic to slow down the bowels. In the chronic forms of diarrhea additional tests must be made, such as a sigmoidoscopy (see page 275) and also a barium enema and possibly an upper GI (gastrointestinal) series. Stool cultures as well as other analytical tests on the stools must be done; then appropriate treatment can be instituted according to the final diagnosis.

How can I prevent diarrhea?

Viral gastroenteritis is difficult to prevent; however, the type of diarrhea that comes from food poisoning such as staphylococcus can be prevented by not allowing dairy products to sit around on a counter but keeping them in the refrigerator. When you travel you can prevent Salmonella or

Shigella diarrhea by not drinking strange water and restricting your intake to wine and beer. If you are going to take the drinking water in the countries that you travel to you should boil it or drink coffee or tea. This will still not prevent you from getting diarrhea from the water that is used to prepare salads, etc. In some countries such as Mexico almost everybody gets diarrhea before they have finished their vacation.

Is diarrhea dangerous?

No, diarrhea is not dangerous, unless it is associated with a malignancy or is a chronic form associated with some other unusual bowel condition. Diarrhea is dangerous in infants.

Dizziness

What is dizziness?

Dizziness can mean a feeling of light-headedness or faintness but most people mention this symptom when they feel that their body or the room around them is turning.

What causes it?

The distinction between light-headedness and a true rotational feeling (vertigo) is very important, because true vertigo usually is due to trouble in the inner ear (semicircular canals) while light-headedness is usually due to trouble in the heart or circulatory system, or else an emotional problem. Motion sickness, labyrinthitis (cold in the inner ear) and Ménière's disease are the most common causes of vertigo, but it may also be due to drugs, tumors or strokes. Some people suffer from vertigo for some time after a concussion (page 133).

The cause of Ménière's disease is not known but it is believed that part of the problem is the accumulation of fluid in the semicircular canals (labyrinth) and "hearing" canals (cochlea). That is why both the balance and hearing are often affected together.

What can I do about it?

You do not have to see your doctor for mild vertigo that does not persist and is not associated with ringing in the ear or loss of hearing and other symptoms. Just simply go to bed and rest for a few days. When the vertigo is severe, persistent, or associated with other symptoms you should see your doctor. He will find the cause and probably prescribe Dramamine and other useful drugs to relieve it. Surgery can be used to treat it but is rarely required.

Is dizziness dangerous?

In most cases dizziness is a harmless symptom and not a sign of a serious disease. Severe vertigo can throw a person to the floor and cause accidents in driving. When dizziness is the sign of a stroke or brain tumor it is more serious, but there are usually other more prominent symptoms to indicate this.

What can I do to prevent it?

If you have a cold, get proper treatment before it spreads to your ears. This usually means bed rest and fluids and decongestants. Don't take drugs indiscriminately that might damage the inner ear such as aspirin in large quantities. Don't smoke or drink excessively and eat a well-balanced diet. Avoid long trips, particularly in a car.

Earache

What is an earache?

An earache is usually an ache in the ear, although some people use the term for just a cracking or ringing in the ear. The important thing to know about an earache is that it is not caused by just one condition but several.

What causes an earache?

An earache may be caused by an infection in the outer, middle or inner ear. Jamming of wax in the ear canal may cause it. It also can be caused simply by blocking of the Eustachian tube (the tube that drains the middle ear into the nose). However the earache is usually caused by an ear infection, most frequently bacterial although it may occasionally be viral. The most common cause of the earache is an infection of the middle ear or otitis media. This infection is usually caused by a bacteria such as streptococcus, pneumococcus, staphylococcus or Klebsiella, but occasionally it is caused by a virus. Almost as frequent as otitis media is otitis externa, or infection of the outer ear, the ear canal. This occurs commonly in kids during the summer when the wax in the outer ear is infected by swimming or the chlorine in the water causes the wax to curdle. Adults get this type of infection from too much wax or too much cleaning of the ear with cotton applicators. Occasionally children may have an earache because of a foreign body in the ear, such as a wad of paper, etc.

What are the symptoms of an earache?

The main symptom of an earache is pain in the ear. In addition there may be draining of the ear and there may be a temperature. Patients who have an infection in the ear associated with or preceded by a cold will have a runny nose and a cough as well.

What can I do about an earache?

The most important thing is to see your doctor. To try to cure your earache yourself is foolish. If your earache is mild it could be simply from a sore throat. In this case it may get better on its own. Do not fool around if it is a severe earache, as this needs immediate medical attention. Your doctor can look into your ear with an otoscope (a light especially designed to illuminate the ear canal) and he can find out if the pain is due to wax, foreign body or infection of the middle or outer ear. He can then prescribe the appropriate antibiotic as well as nose drops or a pill taken by mouth that will cut down the congestion in the ear and nose. If the infection is in the middle ear, ear drops will probably not be of much value unless they have an analgesic (pain relieving agent). Small children may need something to take the temperature down because they may have a very high temperature with this condition. If you catch the earache early it is not often necessary to lance the ear as we used to do in the days before we had antibiotics. Lancing of the ear is not a difficult operation and can be performed fairly painlessly if the proper anesthetic techniques are applied. Don't be alarmed if your doctor decides to put you or your child into the hospital to perform lancing of the ear; it is simply easier to perform this operation under general anesthesia in some patients.

Is an earache dangerous?

No, if it is due to impacted wax in the ear or a foreign body in the ear. If it is due to otitis media, of course, the ear drum can rupture if the infection is allowed to continue.

What will happen if I do not do anything about it?

As I stated, if it is due to infection in the middle ear the ear drum can rupture and you will lose your hearing. Of course today we have ways of repairing the ruptured drum, so it is not as serious as it used to be. However, an infection in the middle ear can spread to involve the inner ear and also to the brain, causing meningitis or a brain abscess. These are the worst complications.

How can I prevent myself from getting an earache?

The best way to prevent yourself from getting an earache is to have periodic examinations by your doctor to make sure you don't have wax. Also, get immediate treatment when you have a cold to prevent the infection in your nose and throat from spreading into your ears. Special methods of prevention must be applied in children who have recurrent ear infections and these will not be dealt with in detail here. Children should wear ear plugs or a nose clip when swimming if they get recurrent ear infections. Also a mother should not clean the wax out of the child's ear vigorously with cotton applicators. For adults I would suggest they do not put anything smaller than their elbow in their ear.

Enlarged Heart

What is an enlarged heart?

I have heard a lot of people say they have an enlarged heart when in reality they don't. Actual enlargement of the heart may be most frequently spotted on an x-ray, and since there are so many of the mobile x-ray units going around the country today, many people are being told that they have enlarged hearts and to report to their family doctor for further evaluation. However, many of these "enlarged hearts" are nothing but a minor or physiological enlargement of the heart and not due to any serious disease.

What causes an enlarged heart?

An enlarged heart may be caused by physiological changes of the heart due to increased work output as in athletes. We commonly refer to this as an athletic heart. But if the enlarged heart is due to actual disease it may be caused by rheumatic fever, congenital heart disease, atherosclerosis, or hypertension. There are a few rare causes that are not necessary to mention in a book like this. The most common cause of an enlarged heart is probably hypertension. Next to that would be rheumatic fever with involvement of the valves of the heart. Atherosclerosis causes enlargement of the heart by causing myocardial infarctions (heart attacks), which when they heal may lead to a weakness in the heart and require the other muscles of the heart to do more work with subsequent hypertrophy.

What are the symptoms and signs of an enlarged heart?

Very few patients actually can tell they have an enlarged heart without a doctor's examination but sometimes they feel their heart contracting or experience palpitations. Occasionally they get shortness of breath and can feel the heart on the left side of the chest or even under the left arm. If the enlarged heart is associated with heart failure then, of course, there will often be fluid in the lungs, ankles and legs.

What can I do about an enlarged heart?

The answer to that is to see your doctor. In many cases no medication will be necessary. If your enlarged heart is due to hypertension he will control your blood pressure. If it is due to heart valve disease or heart failure he may have to give you digitalis to strengthen your heart muscle. Other treatments will be used at his discretion. Don't worry about it! Let the doctor do the worrying!

Fainting Spells

What are fainting spells?

Fainting is the sudden loss of consciousness usually due to a disturbance to the blood supply in the brain, but it may also be due to other causes.

What causes fainting?

The most common cause of fainting is an emotional shock. Bad news about someone's death or about a loved one's illness is sufficient to cause a complete dilation of the blood vessels in the vascular system, causing a pooling of blood in the lower extremities of the body and therefore poor blood supply to the brain. Under these circumstances there is immediate loss of consciousness. But the person regains his consciousness as soon as he is in a recumbent position.

There are many more serious causes of fainting, however. For instance the heart may go into arrest as in Stokes-Adams syndrome; or in an acute heart attack there may be an arrest from ventricular fibrillation. There may be an obstruction of one of the arteries to the brain which will cause a person to black out. Or a sudden loss of blood, as in a ruptured ectopic pregnancy or hemorrhage into the gastrointestinal tract, may cause acute anemia leading to a faint. Epilepsy may cause a faint, in this case without the usual convulsive movements but simply a loss of consciousness. Low blood sugar may cause a fainting spell, most often when a patient has taken an overdose of insulin. Coughing for a long period of time may cause fainting as well. These numerous causes of fainting can be diagnosed by your doctor as soon as he has done a thorough physical examination and evaluation.

To reiterate, the most common cause of fainting is emotional shock; therefore, when you see someone faint in a crowded room do not jump to the conclusion that he has something serious. Another common cause of fainting is simple heat exhaustion. This occurs frequently in crowded rooms, where the temperature is high and a person gets dehydrated, or where the heat causes dilatation of the blood vessels and the person's lowered blood pressure causes him to faint. And some people faint just to get attention.

What are the symptoms and signs of fainting?

Most cases of fainting occur with sweating and a drop in blood pressure; in the common faint due to emotional causes there is a slowing of the heart rate. Prior to the faint the person may feel dizzy and lightheaded and may even feel nauseated. If there is obstruction to one of the arteries of the brain the person may have paralysis of one side of the body associated with the faint.

What can I do about a faint?

The best thing to do is to see your doctor. He will be able to perform the physical examination and the necessary tests to determine the cause of your fainting. Do not postpone visiting the doctor if you have had a fainting spell, because it may be serious.

Is it dangerous?

Most cases of fainting are due simply to emotional causes and are not serious, but only your doctor can determine whether it is serious or not.

How can I prevent fainting?

The common faint due to emotional causes can be prevented by simply avoiding anything which would shock you; however, this is not always possible. In addition avoid crowded, overheated rooms or places where there is not enough oxygen. People who have cardiac or respiratory disorders certainly should avoid crowded rooms or any areas where there would be insufficient oxygen.

Fatigue

What causes fatigue?

One of the most common complaints that my patients come to me with is fatigue. It is rarely due to any disease. The most common cause of fatigue in my practice has been emotional tension. It is very difficult to get people who complain of fatigue to discuss their emotional problems. Most of them deny that they have any emotional problems at all. Some frequent examples of such problems are trouble with a spouse, trouble with a job, suppressed hostility towards a boss, worries about their children's adolescent problems, and worries about in-laws. Consider: if you kept your arms extended and held above your shoulders for any length of time then put them down to a resting position you would experience extreme weakness in those muscles for some time afterward. To a lesser extent every muscle in your body is in a contracted state when you are under emotional tension. At the end of a day of suffering from this emotionally induced muscle tension you are bound to feel tired.

What can I do about emotional fatigue?

The sooner you reveal your real problems to your doctor the sooner you can eliminate this fatigue. Taking tranquilizers is not usually the answer. It may eliminate some of the muscle spasm that is induced by this emotional tension but it will not fully eliminate the fatigue. Occasionally the side effects of the tranquilizers will make you feel more tired. I often cannot establish a good rapport with a patient suffering from fatigue during the first visit; therefore I cannot get down to his emotional problems until he has seen me a few times.

What about other causes of fatigue?

After the patient has denied that he has an emotional problem I usually move to consider other common causes of fatigue. One of the most frequent causes outside of emotion is drinking too much coffee. Some patients drink ten to fifteen cups of coffee a day, and that amount of caffeine can put anybody's body into fatigue by the end of a day. Switching these people over to Sanka or tea will often eliminate the fatigue. Others are smoking too many cigarettes, and nicotine is another drug that will cause increased muscle tension. Contrary to what people might think, nicotine does not relieve emotional tension but only stimulates more emotional tension by exciting all the nerves in your body.

Another common cause of fatigue is drinking. Too much alcohol in the blood relaxes the nervous system at first, but when it wears off there is a state of "hypertension" of all the nerves in the body. Someone who is drinking regularly goes through this day in and day out. In addition the alcohol washes a lot of vitamins out of the blood. A person who drinks too much alcohol is not eating adequately, as a rule, to supply the protein, carbohydrate and fat that the body needs.

With college students the cause of fatigue is often just lack of rest. They often do not get more than three or four hours of sleep a night because they are studying for exams. Their meals are irregular also.

Another common cause of fatigue is improper diet. Many people eat in restaurants, frequently on the run, and their meals are irregular. It is a wonder that they get adequate nutrition. Supplying a one-a-day vitamin in their diet is only half the solution; in addition they must have the essential amino acids in protein foods and the essential fatty acids in fatty foods in order to maintain proper nutrition for the body.

If I have evaluated all the above possibilities without the answer, then I look for diseases that might cause fatigue. One of the most frequent diseases that cause fatigue is anemia, usually due to iron deficiency and usually in women who have heavy menstrual bleeding. Next to that comes hypothyroidism. Fatigue is usually the first sign of hypothyroidism and there are adequate blood tests to check this out immediately. Even if the tests are equivocal I can put the person on a small amount of thyroid to see if his fatigue is relieved. Once these two common diseases are investigated and ruled out one must go further to consider endocrine diseases, such as diabetes mellitus, adrenal insufficiency, hyperthyroidism, menopause, and underactive pituitary glands. Also we must investigate for infection somewhere in the body, such as tuberculosis. Infections do not always cause chills or fever but may gradually eat away the nutrition of the individual. Certain blood disorders, such as leukemia and Hodgkin's disease can, of course, be the cause of fatigue. Occasionally cancer in some part of the body can begin with fatigue without pain or any other symptoms. But I would caution the reader not to jump to the conclusion that he has one of these diseases until he has first looked into his social environment for tension-producing situations. If he has proper insight into his own psychological development and his environment and psychological makeup he can probably eliminate the cause of his fatigue without seeking the help of his physician.

Fever

What is fever?

Fever is an elevated body temperature. Most people run an oral temperature of 98.6°F, but for some a temperature as low as 97.6°F or up to 99.6°F is normal. Everyone's temperature may rise a half a degree or so in the evening. Rectal temperatures are nearly a degree higher.

What causes fever?

Most cases of elevated temperature are due to infectious diseases such as viruses or bacteria. However, almost any disease can cause at least a slight elevation of temperature at one time or another. I have not infrequently seen fever in cancer, heart attacks, and strokes. Rheumatoid arthritis is often asociated with a fever.

What can I do about it?

A moderate temperature (up to 102°) is by itself no cause for alarm unless it persists beyond two or three days. Persistent or high fever warrants prompt consultation with your doctor. In children, the appearance of a rash will usually help distinguish measles and other contagious diseases. Fever associated with a dry cough is usually due to a virus and therefore can be managed with extra fluids, aspirin, and alcohol sponges or a cool bath. When it is caused by a bacteria appropriate antibiotics must be given. Fever with a shaking chill is usually due to a bacterial infection. Next to pneumonia and strep throat, a kidney infection is the most common bacterial cause in adults. If a stiff neck is associated with the fever you should get to the doctor at once as meningitis may have set in.

Is it dangerous?

Since most acute fevers are due to a simple virus they are not serious. With the antibiotics we have today most bacterial infections can be easily cured. Naturally if the fever is due to cancer it is more serious but this can often be dealt with, too.

What can I do to prevent it?

Children should have DPT (diphtheria-pertussis-tetanus), measles, mumps and polio vaccines. Influenza vaccines should be given semiannually to the elderly and people with chronic lung or heart conditions.

Fluid

A common complaint of my patients is that they "have too much fluid in their system." What they usually mean is that they want me to give them a diuretic to get rid of the fluid or loose weight. After a careful physical examination fails to reveal any pathological cause for the fluid I sit down with the patient and discuss just what their fluid comes from. Fluid in a normal person is usually caused by obesity. The fat accumulation allows the fluid to be sucked up into the tissues like a sponge. If the person who has fluid will go on a diet and lose the excess fat the fluid will follow; therefore, a diuretic is nonsense in most people who have fluid. Anyone who takes a diuretic will lose between four and ten pounds but as soon as the diuretic is discontinued this fluid will come right back into the system. It is dangerous for a person without any disease at all to take fluid pills. Fluid pills will cause thickening of the blood and clots in the brain, heart or other areas of the body. I therefore discourage all my patients who upon physical examination show no disease from taking fluid pills. While the use of fluid pills is not as abused as the use of diet pills it certainly runs a close second.

Headaches

What is headache?

A headache is head pain. In this category we must classify diseases of any structure in the head that may cause head pain.

What causes it?

Most commonly headaches are caused by tension of the muscles that suround the head. These may be the muscles in the back of the neck, the muscles in the temple area (the muscles of mastication), or occasionally the muscles of the eyes from eye strain, etc. The second common cause is migraine. This undoubtedly is a hereditary type of headache, because most of these people have family histories of headaches. The other more serious causes of headache, such as brain tumor, are encountered infrequently.

What are the symptoms and signs of a headache?

In contrast to tension headaches, which are steady and dull and usually occur at the end of the day, migraine is a throbbing headache and usually occurs on one side of the head. It may occur on weekends or at the time of the menstrual period. It is not directly related to periods of tension but may follow periods of tension. Recently we have found that migraine is produced by a substance called tyramine in old milk, cheeses and other dairy products, and also in wine. A lot of people refer to migraine as a "sick headache" because it is associated with nausea and vomiting. It is not commonly known that migraine can cause momentary blindness or paralysis of one arm and leg or numbness or tingling in the hands or feet. This is a transient condition and therefore should not alarm the migraine patient. These symptoms do not mean that he is going to get a stroke or any other severe disease.

What can I do about it?

In treating tension headaches it is best to get rid of the tension. There may be tension on the job, problems with the wife or the children, problems with mother or father, or social and economic problems. Sometimes job change or marriage counseling can improve tension headaches. Tranquilizers can often be a great value in preventing these headaches. One can use aspirin or Excedrin to attack the actual tension headache, but it may be necessary to use a narcotic at times. We try to restrain the use of narcotics because these can be habituating.

Recently the treatment of migraine has been more succesful. We can now prevent the attacks with Dilantin, which is also the drug used in epilepsy. Just because your doctor prescribes it in migraine doesn't mean he thinks you have epilepsy. In the past six years a drug called Sansert has been available to prevent the attacks of migraine. Sixty to seventy percent of migraine patients are relieved by either one of these drugs. Sansert occasionally causes untoward side effects. Therefore anyone taking Sansert should be watched carefully by his physician. Dilantin is a very harmless drug in comparison to Sansert. Many attacks have been avoided by restricting the ingestion of dairy products and wine. In many migraine patients psychotherapy and tranquilizers have helped prevent attacks. During the attack we administer a drug that has been around for many years—Cafergot. Some people cannot take this by mouth so they must take the ergotamine in Cafergot by injection.

Many patients with migraine cannot tolerate ergotamine so therefore we must resort to injectable narcotics to relieve the severe attacks. Fortunately most migraine subjects are not prone to addiction; first, because they are often extremely brilliant people with the obsessive-compulsive type of personality; second, because their attacks usually occur only once or twice a month. I have no migraine patients in my practice who are narcotic addicts.

It is important to reassure people who suffer either tension or migraine headaches that they do not have a brain tumor. It is not well known to most lay people that brain tumors are an uncommon cause of headaches and probably the majority of patients with brain tumors do not suffer headaches until they have had several other symptoms.

Next to tension headaches and migraine, probably systemic infections such as viruses or bacteria are the most common cause of headaches. Headaches during measles, mumps, chicken pox or viral influenza should not alarm anyone, but when a headache occurs with a high fever the doctor must always be consulted to make sure the patient does not have meningitis, particularly the youngster. Other important causes of headaches are eyestrain, glaucoma, strabismus (cross-eye), astigmatism, and certain dental conditions such as an abscess or impacted wisdom tooth. Conditions of the nose such as sinusitis and rhinitis, especially from too many cigarettes, may cause headache. Patients should observe from this that in order to have a complete evaluation of a headache it is necessary to see an eye doctor, an ear, nose and throat doctor, and a dentist in addition to your local physician. Your family doctor should be able to advise you on the necessity of consulting these other doctors.

In older people headaches may be due to disease of the cervical (upper) spine, particularly cervical spondylosis. This is a condition in which the discs are degenerated in the cervical spine so that the vertebrae have bony overgrowth and project into the cervical nerve roots compressing them. Since most of the nerves in the skin around the head come from the neck it is understandable that pain in the head is often due to disease of the neck. This type of headache may be improved by wearing a cervical collar, by either heat treatments or ultrasound treatments of the neck, or by traction of the neck.

A common misconception is that headache is often due to hypertension. Actually very few people with hypertension complain of headaches. Headaches due to high blood pressure are located in the sub-occipital (neck) and temporal areas. Amazingly enough, controlling the blood pressure does not always relieve the headache in hypertension.

Are headaches dangerous?

Most headaches are not due to anything serious and are no cause for alarm unless they persist or are associated with other symptoms.

Heartburn

What is heartburn?

By heartburn a patient usually means a burning sensation felt just below the left side of the heart. Heartburn may also occur in the middle of the anterior wall of the chest, the mid-epigastrium or hypochondrium. This may be increased by swallowing, deep breathing or exercise. It may occur in association with meals or it may have no association with meals. It often awakens the patient from sleep at night.

What causes heartburn?

Heartburn is not a burn of the heart! Heartburn almost invariably is due to some sort of disease of the esophagus, particularly the lower esophagus. The most common disease of the esophagus causing heartburn is *esophagitis,* an inflammation of the esophagus produced by reflux of acid from the stomach into the esophagus. Esophagitis is often associated with a hiatal hernia. A *hiatal hernia* is a widening of the normal hole in the diaphragm that allows the esophagus to pass through to the stomach. If this hole is very wide the stomach may herniate up through the diaphragm into the chest. Under these circumstances there is poor closure of the sphincter between the esophagus and stomach. Therefore acid can leak backwards from the stomach into the esophagus and burn it very easily. Of course the esophagus may be burned by other things, particularly food that is too cold or too hot and alcoholic or carbonated beverages. Heartburn may also come from actual disease of the heart, such as pericarditis, but this is very unusual. Patients sometimes say they have heartburn when they actually have a neuritis, a disease of the upper part of the back, or disease of the gall bladder. A lot of people think they have gall stones when they have heartburn but this is not likely. True heartburn is also not usually caused by a gastric or duodenal ulcer.

What can I do about it?

If you have a persistent heartburn consult your physician. He will perform blood tests, x-rays of your gastrointestinal tract, and probably an electrocardiogram. If these are negative he may actually look down into your stomach and esophagus with a light called a gastroscope or esophagoscope. If you don't do anything about heartburn, chances are it will never cause you any severe problem. However, there is some evidence that severe esophagitis, the major cause of heartburn, can cause spasm of the coronary arteries in the heart. Therefore it is wise to get the esophagitis cured so that this will be less likely. In treating esophagitis there are five different things that we usually prescribe. First, we elevate the head of the bed on six- to eight-inch blocks, so that during the night the acid in the stomach does not leak up into the esophagus. Second, we tell the patient to refrain from eating food that is too hot or too cold and alcoholic or carbonated beverages. Third, we put the patient on antacids, such as Maalox or milk of magnesia, etc., and give them a bland diet that does not contain much spice or stomach irritants. Fourth, since it is important not to eat too much at one time, we divide the meals up into six small feedings a day. Fifth, tight girdles and other tight apparel are prohibited. If these conservative measures do not cure the esophagitis, surgery must be performed to either close the hernia or at least create a better sphincter between the esophagus and the stomach.

Heart Murmurs

What is a heart murmur?

A heart murmur is a rubbing or humming sound heard over the heart. This can be heard with the ear placed on the chest or with a stethoscope. It is produced by the turbulence of blood as it goes through the heart. In this sense if we listen carefully with highly sensitive instruments almost everybody would have a heart murmur because the blood produces some turbulence in every heart as it passes through. At least fifty percent of heart murmurs that can be heard with a stethoscope are not due to disease.

What causes a heart murmur?

As I said above a heart murmur is usually caused by turbulence in the heart as the blood rushes through. What increases the turbulence in the heart is disease of the heart valves in many cases. There are four major valves: the tricuspid, pulmonic, mitral and aortic. In rheumatic or congenital heart disease these valves may be tight or scarred and become fixed in position at times so that the turbulence of the blood as it rushes through them is increased. Sometimes the valves become so narrow that only a trickle of blood can get through with each heart beat. In other cases the valves become fixed in an open position so that they fail to close with each heart beat at the proper time. Heart murmurs are also produced by dilatation of the heart, which separates the valve leaves from each other. Diseases on the outside of the heart cause murmurs as the heart contracts against other structures in the chest cage. If there is inflammation on the outside of the heart then there is sometimes a rubbing between the two layers of the outside of the heart called the pericardium.

Heart murmurs can also be produced by dilatations or distortions of the main vessels that come to and from the heart; thus an aneurysm of the aorta (the main artery leading from the heart) can cause murmurs.

What are the symptoms and signs of a heart murmur?

There are hardly any symptoms from a heart murmur. Occasionally a heart murmur may be so loud that the patient can actually hear it but this is very unusual. If the murmur is due to severe disease of the valves the heart becomes enlarged and the patient may feel palpitations of the heart. He may feel the enlarged heart in his chest, but this is not too common either. If there is associated heart failure he develops shortness of breath, blue lips and often swollen ankles and legs.

What can I do about a heart murmur?

In many cases your heart murmur is not due to any disease so there is nothing to be done about it. You should lead a normal life and not worry about it. However, if your doctor feels that your heart murmur is due to disease, then you must discover whether it is rheumatic fever, congenital heart disease or arteriosclerosis, and treat it. In most cases pathological heart murmurs are due to rheumatic heart disease. If the valves that are diseased by rheumatic heart disease become too narrowed or too dilated they must be repaired surgically. It will be up to your doctor to decide this when the time arises. Until that time if he tells you that you can lead a normal life, please do! Do not harbor unrealistic fears about a heart murmur that restrict your work and play.

What will happen if I don't do anything about a heart murmur?

As I said before, you can frequently do very little because in many cases it is a functional (normal) murmur. If your heart murmur is due to disease of your valves you must get frequent checks with your doctor so that he can see whether the valve disease is getting worse, or whether the valve is not closing properly, or whether the valve is actually becoming fixed so that it does not allow very much blood to pass through.

How can I prevent myself from getting a murmur?

The best way to prevent yourself from getting a murmur is to keep from getting streptococcal infections. These occur in crowded areas such as theaters, school rooms or churches. Since it is pretty impossible to avoid going to these areas I'm sure very few of you will practice this prevention. However, it has been found that people who are on poor diets, or who are fatigued or overworked also get these infections frequently; and these are conditions you can correct. It has been found that these infections are more common in poorer areas of town; in the wealthier suburban areas the incidence is much less. Good general health habits are most important in avoiding rheumatic fever. Prompt treatment of a sore throat (due to streptococcus) with penicillin will also prevent rheumatic fever. Patients who have had one attack of rheumatic fever should remain on prophylactic penicillin indefinitely. The prevention of hypertension and atherosclerosis is discussed in pages 78, 182.

High Blood Pressure

What is high blood pressure?

High blood pressure is the elevation of your blood pressure (as recorded by a special instrument called a *sphygmomanometer*) above the levels generally accepted as normal by the medical profession. These levels may vary with the age, but between the ages of fifteen and fifty the accepted levels are 140/90. Usually when your doctor tells you what your blood pressure is he gives you only the systolic pressure, or the upper pressure. However, in discussing high blood pressure, or *hypertension* as it is called in medical circles, the lower pressure is much more important. The upper pressure can vary from one day to the next quite a bit due to emotional stress and other factors. An elevation of your lower pressure—if it is *consistent*—almost invariably means a definite pathological constriction or hardening of your small arteries, the arterioles.

What causes high blood pressure?

Almost every American has experienced high blood pressure at one time or another, particularly an elevation of their upper pressure—the systolic pressure. However, at least ten to twenty percent of Americans have high blood pressure due to pathological causes. In most of these cases the cause is unknown and therefore is classified as *essential hypertension.* This form of hypertension is usually due to heredity or other constitutional factors. In at least ten percent of the cases of hypertension, however, the cause of the elevation of blood pressure is a disease of one organ or another. Commonly it is the kidneys, which may be diseased by infection (pyelonephritis); by an allergic reaction, as in glomerulonephritis; or by obstruction, as might occur with a stone or a constriction of the ureter, the tube that leads from the kidney. The adrenal gland may also be the cause of hypertension, especially tumors of the adrenal gland. (This should not make everyone who reads this think his hypertension is due to a tumor of the adrenal gland.) There are also a couple of conditions of the heart that can produce hypertension, such as rheumatic heart disease with aortic insufficiency (a leak of the aortic valve), and also coarctation of the aorta, which is a congenital constriction of the main artery that leads from the heart.

I think there is too much concern over the level of a person's blood pressure. Patients expect their blood pressure to be taken every time they come to the doctor's office, and, while they may be feeling perfectly well when they come in, if they find that their pressure is high they immediately feel sick. This is ridiculous! As I stated above, your pressure may vary from day to day so much that to be worried over a single reading is foolish. Also what is normal for one person may be abnormal for another. I find many of my patients over seventy have blood pressures of 170 mm. or 180 mm. and I do not believe they require treatment. It is more important in our examination that we look at the arteries at the back of the eye and listen to the heart and evaluate the kidneys by a urine test in determining whether your hypertension is cause for alarm. I know of many patients who have had high elevations of their blood pressure for ten to fifteen years without any evidence of enlargement of their heart or a secondary disease in their kidneys. These patients rarely develop any serious complications, and they would certainly get more complications from worrying about the high blood pressure than they would from the high blood pressure itself. So, for the patient who has a high blood pressure his worst fear could be from fear itself.

What are the symptoms and signs of high blood pressure?

Aside from the elevated pressure reading, you may have headaches, blurred vision, dizziness, nausea, fatigue and occasionally chest pain or swollen ankles.

What can I do about high blood pressure?

If you have a consistent elevation of blood pressure the first thing I do is make sure that there is not a condition of the kidneys or the adrenal gland causing this. This involves certain tests including the intravenous pyelogram (a special x-ray with dye injected into the vein to show the kidneys), and a special twenty-four-hour urine sample to look for hormones (from the adrenal gland) that might be causing high blood pressure. If a tumor of the adrenal gland is found surgery is the answer to treatment. However in the majority of patients no cause of the hypertension can be found in the kidneys, the adrenal gland, or other areas, and these patients are treated with drugs.

The first drug that we use is a good water pill or diuretic. These pills are not given to take the water out of the system but to remove the salt, which is known to be elevated in the body of a hypertensive patient. This will often bring the blood pressure back to normal without any other medication. However, if this is unsuccessful then drugs that actually lower the blood pressure directly must be used. I make mention of only a few of these, such as reserpine, Apresoline, and Ismelin, but your doctor knows best which of these drugs you can tolerate and which would be most appropriate for your individual case. In some cases tranquilizers alone will bring the pressure back to normal. If your weight is elevated you should get this down to normal as this too will often cure the high blood pressure. Restriction of salt today is not as important as it used to be, because the "water pill" or diuretic removes the extra salt from your system. Anything in your life that can be done to remove tension should be done. You should see your doctor frequently for evaluation of your blood pressure because sometimes it can creep up. He will want to check a urine sample and do an electrocardiogram from time to time to see what effect the hypertension is having on your body.

Is high blood pressure dangerous?

If you follow your doctor's orders and your doctor's prescription regularly and do not throw the drugs away or take them irregularly, then there is no reason why you cannot live a long and happy life with hypertension.

Jaundice

What is jaundice?

Jaundice is a yellowing of the skin and eyes due to backing up of bile from the liver or accumulation of it in the blood stream. After the bile gets into the blood stream it is absorbed into the skin.

What causes it?

Jaundice may be caused by hepatitis, gall bladder trouble, cancer of the pancreas, cancer of any of the ducts draining the liver and cancer of the liver. It may be caused by an increase in breakdown of blood which cannot be adequately handled by the liver and gall ducts and acumulates in the blood as a result. A good example of a condition causing this is sickle-cell anemia.

What can I do about it?

Your physician will run several diagnostic tests to determine whether you have hepatitis or one of the other conditions mentioned above. Then he will administer the appropriate treatment, whether it be surgery for gall stones or cancer, or whether it be for your blood condition.

Is it dangerous?

Jaundice is a very dangerous thing if it is left untreated. It is a sure sign that you should see your physician. Some very famous people have died from the ravages of hepatitis.

If the jaundice is due to gall stones or cancer in the biliary tract or the pancreas, it is of course even more serious.

How can I prevent myself from getting it?

Of course the prevention of jaundice from cancer is pretty difficult, but prevention of jaundice from gall stones is not difficult since you can get the gall stones removed if you know that you have them. To prevent yourself from getting hepatitis you should make sure that you drink clean water and stay away from poorly cooked seafood such as clams. Make sure that you eat in clean restaurants. Make sure that all your foods are cooked properly.

Low Blood Pressure

It is very surprising to me that many patients who come to my office have been diagnosed as having low blood pressure by other physicians and have actually been given treatment for this condition. The vast majority of these people are normal and have no low blood pressure. Yet they insist that they have received a great deal of improvement from the medicine that was prescribed for the low blood pressure.

What is low blood pressure?

Just as with high blood pressure low blood pressure in one patient may not be low blood pressure in another patient. In general a patient may be considered to have low blood pressure if the systolic, or upper, reading on the blood pressure recording device is below 90 mm. The lower reading may vary anywhere from 40 to 60 or 70, but most physicians do not mention this pressure to the patient. With some patients a systolic pressure of 80 or 85 is normal. Children up to fifteen years of age normally have a pressure in the 70 to 90 mm. range. During pregnancy a pressure between 80 and 90 mm. may be considered normal.

What causes low blood pressure?

If low blood pressure is truly due to a disease it may be from anemia, tuberculosis, or from dehydration or loss of salt from the body as occurs in the hot summer months. It may be from adrenal insufficiency (a decreased output of hormones from the adrenal gland). It may also be due to some type of heart condition. A sudden drop in blood pressure may be due to a heart attack from coronary occlusion (obstruction of the coronary artery). Low blood pressure can also be due to acute bleeding, whether it is internal or external through a cut or wound. Some people get an acute drop of blood pressure from a simple faint, as when they see something that causes a great deal of fear or causes a sickening feeling through their body.

What can I do about my low blood pressure?

If your family physician has checked you over carefully and found none of these unusual causes of low blood pressure and you are feeling good except for the fact that someone told you that you have a low pressure, there is actually no treatment necessary. Your low pressure is probably normal for you. However, if he does discover one of these conditions obviously immediate treatment is warranted. Rarely a person has fainting spells or other symptoms that can be attributed to low blood pressure in the absence of any other conceivable cause. In this case you must take a drug to elevate the pressure so that you stop having fainting spells. Frequently people who have this type of low blood pressure have a psychological problem, and referral to a psychiatrist would be in order if the family physician cannot pinpoint the emotional problem. In general, then, low blood pressure without any symptoms is no cause for alarm and no treatment is necessary. A good thorough checkup is in order if low blood pressure is discovered to rule out the other diseases that may be causing it.

Lumbago and Other Back Pain

What is lumbago?

Lumbago is really a lay term that indicates a pain in the back, usually the lower back.

What causes it?

Low back pain can be ascribed to almost one hundred different causes, but it is most commonly due to poor posture. I find so many people slump in their chairs or slump while they are driving that it is a wonder there is not more back pain from bad posture. As I have said elsewhere in this book, soft mattresses are another cause for chronic low back pain. If people would do daily exercises of their back muscles there would be much less lumbago.

Of the various diseases that cause low back pain probably the most common ones are osteoarthritis (see page 113) and herniated disc (see page 185). Osteoarthritis of the back is usually due to constant weight bearing, pressure or trauma causing overgrowth of bone at the joints of the back, and calcium deposits. A herniated disc is the rupture of the material in the center of one of the little cushions (disc) that lie between each of the vertebrae in the back. This material extrudes into the nerves that run through the spine causing pain not only in the back but often down one or both legs. The pain down the legs is called *sciatica.* This symptom distinguishes herniated disc from the more common causes of back pain, such as poor posture and osteoarthritis. In menopause the loss of calcium in the vertebrae causes back pain. This is probably secondary to the lack of estrogen in the body. Other causes of back pain are curvature of the spine, congenital deformities, tumors, other types of arthritis such as rheumatoid arthritis or gouty arthritis, and pelvic tumors (such as uterine fibroids, etc.). Women of child-bearing age get back pain when they are pregnant, and they also get a lot of back pain associated with their periods. The exact cause of this is not certain, but it may be due to a loosening of the ligaments caused by the change in hormonal balance or it may be referred from a spasm of the womb.

What can I do about lumbago?

Probably the most important thing to do before consulting your physician is to make sure that you have good posture and that you have a good mattress. If you have persistent back pain and both of these possibilities are ruled out, then have your physician examine you. He may find that you have sciatica or other signs of compression of the nerves in your back that would indicate a herniated disc. If he x-rays your back he may discover other causes, such as arthritis, tumors, or a curvature. By a pelvic examination he may discover some cause in your womb.

Is it dangerous?

Intermittent back pain itself is not dangerous, but a persistent back pain should alert you to a possible serious condition, in which case you should have an examination, not by a chiropractor but a medical doctor. A herniated disc is not a serious thing unless it is causing compression of the nerves enough to paralyze the legs. One can live with a herniated disc for years without needing surgery.

Lumps in the Breast

What causes a lump in the breast?

Lumps in the breast, contrary to what most lay people believe, are most commonly benign and not cancerous. A lump in the breast may be the result of enlargement of one of the glands that secrete milk, or it may be enlargement of one of the lymph glands in the breast. Occasionally a lump in the breast is due to the walling off of a portion of the gland causing a cyst with fluid inside of it. But one should not hesitate to consult her physician when she finds a lump in her breast. Many lumps in the breast must be considered cancerous until proven otherwise. Cancer is most likely when there is an associated discharge of blood or mucous from the nipple and some deformity of the breast.

What can I do about a lump in the breast?

The most important thing is to report to your physician as soon as you have discovered a lump in your breast. He can determine whether other tests need to be performed or whether it is just a benign condition. Sometimes he will have you come back in two to three weeks for a reexamination before he proceeds with further diagnostic procedures. He will often order an x-ray called mammography to help determine whether the lump is malignant or not. If he is still in doubt then you will be scheduled for surgery and a biopsy immediately.

Is it dangerous?

A lump in the breast is considered dangerous until you have been examined by your physician and told that it is nothing to worry about.

How can I prevent lumps from coming into my breast?

There is really little that you can do to prevent lumps in the breast. However the use of birth control pills in the last ten years has contributed to a greater incidence of benign lumps in the breast. Birth control pills are not *known* to contribute to cancer of the breast at this point. There is no known cause of cancer of the breast as yet.

Nosebleeds

What causes nosebleeds?

Nosebleeds are very common in children and adults. They are due to numerous causes, but the most frequent cause is a local inflammation of a small area in the front of the nose called "Little's area." In this area blood vessels are very numerous and very close to the surface of the nasal mucosa. Probably the most common cause of nosebleeds in kids is picking the nose. Apparently in both kids and adults this little area becomes inflamed by rhinitis, hay fever, and severe colds. Nosebleeds are rarely due to a defect in the clotting of the blood such as hemophilia. In adults other common causes are hypertension, asthma and heart disease. In children one of the first signs of rheumatic fever may be a nosebleed. Older adults who have frequent nosebleeds should have a thorough examination by an ear, nose and throat specialist for cancer, particularly older adults who smoke.

What can I do about a nosebleed?

The most important thing to do the first time you get a nosebleed is to squeeze your nose or apply a clothespin over the end of your nose. The nose clips that kids use when they are swimming can be used. If these are applied for five minutes most nosebleeds will be stopped, as ninety percent are due to the bleeding in "Little's area" in the front of the inner nose. It is better for a person with a nosebleed to sit up, contrary to previous belief that the person should lie down. If you bend forward each time you release pressure the blood will come out of the front of the nose rather than going down the back of the throat unnoticed. If conservative measures like this do not work it may be necessary to go to your doctor and have your nose packed. He may apply a coagulating agent to the area of bleeding. If the nosebleed is very severe he must pack the nose from back to front. There are several drugs that he can give by injection to help your nosebleeds stop, such as vitamin K and estrogen substances. He will check your blood pressure and if it is high bring it down with some anti-hypertensive drugs. Usually a diagnostic work-up is not necessary if you have had one nosebleed, but if you have repeated nosebleeds then you must undergo this thorough investigation.

What will happen if you don't do anything about it?

Usually the nosebleed will stop after you have bled a while. In most cases your body can regenerate the blood you have lost and you will have suffered no serious consequences. This is why it is silly to call a doctor at the first nosebleed; but if they persist then you must see a doctor.

Obesity

What is obesity?

Obesity is overweight or an excess of fat in relation to the other tissues of your body (muscle, bone, etc.). Insurance companies have compiled a chart of the average weight for each height and body build, but if you are within ten pounds of these you are not overweight. Obesity may be a symptom or a disease in itself.

What causes it?

A few cases of obesity may be due to glandular trouble, such as underactive thyroid or overactive adrenal gland. About five to ten percent of cases of obesity are due to heredity. However most obesity is due to relative or absolute overeating. In other words, if your intake of food is greater than your output of energy then you will gain weight. Why do people overeat? Nine times out of ten it is because of anxiety, depression, or lack of will power and motivation to stay thin.

What can I do about it?

Of course the simple answer is "stop eating." But if this is all diet specialists told their patients they would be out of business. The best-known treatments are the diet pills, such as amphetamines and their derivatives. Diet specialists have other drugs to help you reduce. They actually do depress the appetite, but their effect may wear off in six to eight weeks unless therapy is interrupted for a week. The amphetamines stimulate the nervous system so that they may relieve any associated depression or fatigue. Newer amphetamines have a less stimulating effect and are less likely to cause a rapid heart rate and high blood pressure than the original ones. Recently Ionamin (R) has been introduced as an appetite depressant without any stimulating effects at all. It has proven to be very effective in my practice.

There are three other forms of therapy in the physician's armory that are much more important than diet pills. These are diets, psychotherapy, and tranquilizers. There are almost as many reducing diets as there are physicians, because in order for a diet to be successful it must be tailored to the individual's needs and tastes. The "simplest" are the low-calorie diets; but they leave the patient hungry and are difficult to follow because you must measure portions carefully. Many people eat in restaurants today and must refer to a calorie book before ordering; they can't weigh the portions individually.

I prefer to prescribe a diet that simply excludes foods with a lot of calories and fat. I call this the "fruit and vegetable diet," although it includes crackers and no-calorie or low-calorie beverages (tea, coffee, etc.) as well. We in America are "poisoned" every day because our diets are largely carnivorous, or animal rather than vegetable. Have you ever seen a fat vegetarian? I haven't. That's why my diet eliminates all meat, milk and milk products. Also I eliminate potatoes, pastries, and wheat products (except crackers), because they are high in calories. I often allow my patients who do not wish to lose fast to eat fish and chicken. But for those who will tolerate the "fruit and vegetable diet" there is a special reward. They can eat anything they want one day a week, preferably Sunday. This gives them the courage to go on. It says in the Bible that "six days shalt thou labor" and on the seventh day you rest. That's the principle of the reward. There is another important principle of this diet compared to a low-calorie diet. On low-calorie diets you lose by losing the fat out of the fat cells. The fat cell, however, may not be destroyed: therefore, when you start eating normally again the fat is drawn right up into the cell like a sponge. You may regain all you lost if you don't continue to count calories closely. Since my diet largely eliminates protein and cholesterol—the components of the fat-cell wall and nucleus—the fat cell will usually be destroyed along with the fat. When you resume a normal diet you will stay thin more consistently. This theory is not proven but makes good sense.

Psychotherapy begins when you visit the physician. The simple act of making visits to your physician regularly while you reduce is a form of psychotherapy. It builds a relationship with someone else who is concerned about your weight, someone who understands you and can sympathize with you. However, some patients need a physician to bawl them out or demand that they lose weight. Others cooperate better with a sympathetic approach. Both these methods remotivate the patient. There are other ways to motivate the patient. For example, a husband who doesn't care about his wife's weight may be educated to show concern; and a husband who is always complaining about his wife's weight may be educated to get off her back. There must be a happy medium. I have remotivated many patients by pointing out the dangers of obesity: it contributes to high blood pressure, heart trouble, diabetes and many other diseases; it makes you a great surgical risk; and it contributes to more accidental injuries.

Some of my patients are motivated to lose because they want me or someone else to see how beautiful they can look if they are thin. When the husband begins avoiding sexual relations they hope they can change things by reducing. Financial or social reward may remotivate the patient. For example, an Air Force nurse was able to reduce because she was told she could not be promoted to colonel unless she did. Many women reduce so that they can fit into their favorite clothes, others so that their husband will buy them a fur coat.

I motivate patients financially by reducing the office fee each time they show progress and increasing it if they don't. Sometimes there are deep-seated emotional problems that require long-term psychotherapy. For example, one patient was so restricted as a child that the only thing her parents didn't scold her about was eating; in fact they highly approved of it. When she was fully grown and her calorie requirements leveled off, she couldn't stop eating. Another patient began to eat because she found sex with her husband a bore and figured obesity would make him leave her alone. I could name many other examples.

Because overeating is often caused by anxiety or depression, tranquilizers and antidepressants can be extremely valuable in helping patients reduce. Many forms of depression are not psychological but physiological. Therefore, I believe drug therapy is the only solution. I use Librium and Valium for anxiety and Elavil or Sinequan for depression; there are many other useful drugs. Certain drugs, however, should not be used to reduce. Water pills are useless and may cause harm by raising the blood sugar and uric acid (causing gout). Digitalis is dangerous, and therefore it is now unlawful to prescribe it for obesity. Thyroid tablets can be used where laboratory tests show an underactive thyroid.

Your physician knows when and how to use all these therapeutic methods to help you reduce. It is difficult to do it alone.

Is obesity dangerous?

This question was already answered affirmatively above. Besides contributing to many diseases, surgical risks and accidents, obesity is psychologically disturbing.

How can I prevent it?

By eating a well-balanced diet, between 1500 and 2500 calories, taking a daily vitamin supplement and regular exercise you can usually beat the rap. However, restriction of liquor and regularity of meals are also important. If you overeat because of emotional problems it is wise to discuss these with your physician before you become obese.

Palpitations

What are palpitations?

"Palpitations" usually signifies rapid or irregular beating of the heart. The term can, however, represent fluttering of the diaphragm or abdominal muscles. Some patients call palpitation a "fluttering" or "jumping" of the heart.

What causes them?

Palpitations are caused by anything that stimulates the heart. Usually they are due to fear or anxiety and excessive smoking or coffee consumption. Eating a heavy meal or having one drink too many may cause them too. Irregular beating of the heart usually signifies a serious heart condition, such as damage to the muscle wall (myocardial infarction) or congestion of the heart, or an overactive thyroid or drug intoxication. One condition associated with a very rapid heart beat is usually innocuous; that is paroxysmal auricular tachycardia. It is usually brought on by nerves and can be easily treated by your physician. It rarely causes permanent damage.

What can I do about palpitations?

If you're suffering from palpitations without any other symptoms, cut down on coffee and cigarettes and they will probably disappear. If you are very nervous, see your friend, a minister, or a psychiatrist and get to the root of the problem. If none of these causes applies to you, then see your physician. He will run a series of diagnostic tests, including a cardiogram, to determine the cause and begin treatment.

What will happen if I don't do anything about them?

Nothing will happen in most cases if you have no other symptoms. However, if you have pain in the chest or shortness of breath, you will probably get a heart attack eventually.

What can I do to prevent them?

This has already been answered above.

Rash

What is a rash?

A rash is a breaking out of the skin. It may be red, brownish, or white in color; and the lesions may be flat, raised like a pimple, scaly, blister-like, or pus pockets. The rash can be focal or generalized.

What causes it?

The most common rash we see is contact dermatitis. This may be due to detergents, poison ivy, hair sprays, cosmetics, dogs, cats, or even various fabrics. The next most common cause is atopic dermatitis, or eczema. This is usually hereditary and begins in childhood. Acne (page 105), psoriasis (page 226), and athlete's foot are other common causes. Contagious diseases such as measles used to be common causes of skin rash and still are seen often. A rash may be associated with rheumatic fever, typhoid fever, and many bacterial and viral infections. It is also seen in blood diseases and occasionally in cancer.

What can I do about it?

Most rashes if left alone will go away by themselves. Rashes associated with measles and other contagious diseases are of this nature. The miraculous drug cortisone has been a revolution in clearing up most rashes. Your doctor will prescribe it in a cream, ointment or lotion and if the rash is more generalized it can be given by mouth or injection. Athlete's foot can be cured with Tinactin, available without a prescription.

Is it dangerous?

Rashes by themselves are not dangerous. If they become infected they may constitute a threat. Rashes can be the sign of a more serious condition, such as a form of meningitis, a bacterial infection of the heart, a blood disease or cancer.

What can I do to prevent it?

Avoid contactants and skin irritants. Don't bathe too much. If you have an allergy get skin tests to find out what the cause is so that you can avoid it. Poison ivy shots are useful. Measles vaccines should be given to all children.

Rectal Bleeding

What causes rectal bleeding?

Rectal bleeding is most commonly caused by hemorrhoids or a crack in the skin around the rectum, called a rectal fissure. But it may be a sign of cancer of the rectum or anywhere in the gastrointestinal tract. Other causes of rectal bleeding are colitis, ulcers, and bacterial and parasitic infection of bowels.

What can I do about it?

Rectal bleeding after one or two bowel movements is nothing to worry about and you may delay calling your doctor. However, if it persists for more than three or four days, you should see your doctor. He will examine you with a sigmoidoscope (page 275) and a barium enema (x-ray of the bowels) to determine the exact cause and treat accordingly.

What will happen if I don't do anything about it?

In most cases nothing, because it is usually due to a fissure or hemorrhoid. However, if it is due to cancer your life is in danger because by the time you get other symptoms it may have spread too far to remove surgically.

How can I prevent rectal bleeding?

Hemorrhoids (page 183) and rectal fissures, the most common causes of rectal bleeding, can be prevented by having regular bowel movement. If you are constipated, do not strain. Lubricate the rectum with Vaseline before the movement or use a tap water or Fleets enema. Add more vegetables and fruit to your diet.

Sterility and Infertility

What are sterility and infertility?

Both terms signify the inability to conceive or have children, but usually a patient is labeled sterile when a physical cause can be found and labeled infertile when no physical cause is found. For example, a man who produces a normal number of sperm but can't penetrate his wife will not have children but is not sterile. He is infertile.

What causes them?

Sterility may be caused by failure to make eggs or sperm, blockage of the tubes (that carry eggs to the womb or sperm to the penis), or imperfect lining of the womb during the menstrual cycle. It may also be caused by glandular trouble such as hypothyroidism (underactive thyroid). Other rarer causes will not be dealt with here. Infertility may be caused by sterility but also by psychological or social problems.

What can I do about them?

A proper diet and good clean living are important. If you have emotional problems, talk to a professional and straighten them out. You really should not delay seeing a doctor, because something simple, such as inflammation of the womb, may be cleaned up easily. Fifty percent of women can be helped with this problem but only five percent of men.

Are they dangerous?

No. However it is a tremendous psychological burden once you begin thinking you are sterile. Go to your doctor and find out the truth. If you are, he will know how to help you bear the burden.

What can I do to prevent sterility or infertility?

Stay away from x-rays and venereal disease. Don't hold anger or anxiety in! Discuss it with someone. Get regular physical checkups and good nutrition.

"Tired Blood" (Anemia)

What is "tired blood"?

You have all heard the advertisements on television about "tired blood." What these really refer to is anemia. These advertisements ignore the fact that today most people get a very good diet containing enough iron to make it unnecessary to add additional iron. Nevertheless there are people who are anemic.

Anemia means that a person has insufficient blood cells to carry the oxygen required for his body. Some anemic people have sufficient blood cells but do not have enough iron in their blood cells.

What causes anemia?

Anemia has many causes but the most common cause is iron deficiency. This may result from an improper diet or, more importantly, from loss of blood from the body. Women are subject to this more than men because they have periodic menstruation. Women lose 100 to 200 cc's of blood every month. Sometimes they lose a great deal more than that, so that their diet cannot give them enough iron to compensate for this blood loss. Most often the excessive blood loss is simply due to changing of hormones in the woman's body, but sometimes it is due to a fibroid tumor of her womb, a miscarriage, or other things. Both men and women may lose a lot of blood from an ulcer in the stomach or duodenum. Other conditions of the gastrointestinal tract that may make them lose blood are ulcerative colitis, hemorrhoids, and diverticuli. Infants who come from the ghettos are most likely to have anemia as a result of a poor diet. However, if these people pay attention to the television commercials they do not have the money to purchase the various things advertised to cure "tired blood." Some other forms of anemia are due to hereditary disorders (sickle-cell anemia, Mediterranean anemia, etc.). Sickle-cell anemia occurs in Negroes, and in this type of anemia all the iron or all other medicine in the world will be of very little help. Mediterranean anemia is found most often in people with Italian or Greek ancestry. Here again nutrition is not going to help restore the blood to normal. Older people develop a type of anemia called pernicious anemia, which is due to the body's inability to absorb vitamin B_{12} from the diet because the stomach no longer produces the proper enzyme to absorb B_{12}. When an older person develops tired blood it can be from either blood loss or this factor. However, pernicious anemia may occur in people of all ages.

What are the symptoms and signs of "tired blood"?

Probably the most important symptom is fatigue, but anemic people may also suffer headaches, weight loss and loss of appetite. Anemic women may start menstruating more heavily; this is ironic in view of the fact that they have less blood in their bodies. Other symptoms include numbness and tingling in the hands and feet and difficulty sleeping. The doctor will notice a pallor of the skin, nails, and eyelids long before the patient notices it. In those cases where the anemia is due to blood loss the patient will see black tarry stools or may even vomit blood. The hereditary forms of anemia may be present with an acute anemia accompanied by pallor and jaundice because of the excessive breakdown of the red cells. In these cases there may be fever as well. There are many other symptoms of anemia that are too numerous to mention in this writing.

What can I do about anemia?

The most important thing to do is to insure that your diet has the basic seven foods and adequate amounts of iron. Spinach alone is not necessary. If there are enough eggs in the diet one will get enough iron. Also many of the green vegetables contain significant amounts of iron. There is no harm for a woman, particularly of child-bearing age, to take an iron supplement, either separately or in a multivitamin pill. This is good common sense. However, it is unnecessary for women beyond the age of menstruation. I think it is valuable to take a good one-a-day vitamin, as this will improve the general nutrition in addition to preventing anemia.

If you notice that you're losing a lot of blood during your periods or if you have black stools you should immediately consult your physician. He will be able to determine the cause of the excessive blood loss. If your main symptom is fatigue and you think that you have "tired blood" or anemia, do not expect that the doctor will find anemia every time. There are many, many causes of fatigue. If you have pernicious anemia B_{12} shots given by your family physician will suffice to correct the condition; however all the B_{12} in the world *taken by mouth* will *not* cure pernicious anemia. There are a lot of doctors that give B_{12} for fatigue in general, without a clear-cut diagnosis of pernicious anemia. I know of no other condition that B_{12} actually cures besides pernicious anemia, but nevertheless I have found in my experience that people with nervous disorders do improve with injections of B_{12}. It is understandable, therefore, that doctors use these injections if only for the psychological value.

What will happen if I don't do anything about it?

If the anemia becomes severe you will not get enough oxygen into your body and you will go into shock and die.

But in mild anemias your body can compensate, often for years. Very few people die from primary anemia, if they are under the care of a physician.

Vaginal Bleeding

What is vaginal bleeding?

Vaginal bleeding is the passing of blood through the vagina. Of course in women of menstrual age (between ten and fifty) it is normal to have vaginal bleeding every twenty-four to thirty-five days. This bleeding usually is not enough to saturate more than four or five tampons or sanitary napkins a day and rarely contains any large clots. Abnormal vaginal bleeding is bleeding that continues beyond the seven days of the menstrual period or between the menstrual periods. It may be a small amount of black or brownish material or profuse bright red bleeding with clots.

What is the cause of vaginal bleeding?

The most common cause of vaginal bleeding, whether it is bleeding in between periods or an increased amount of bleeding at the time of the period, is dysfunctional uterine bleeding. This means that it is due to an alteration in hormone secretion during the cycle. Dysfunctional uterine bleeding is very common in women around the menopause and puberty. This is why it is silly for any woman who has abnormal vaginal bleeding to get too worried. Other causes are endometrial hyperplasia (overgrowth of the lining of the womb), fibroids, and polyps in the lining of the womb. These are not malignant. An underactive thyroid or anemia may cause vaginal bleeding.

Most women with vaginal bleeding think they have cancer. It is true that cancer of the mouth or lining of the womb, such as a carcinoma of the cervix, may cause vaginal bleeding but these are not the usual causes of vaginal bleeding during the child-bearing years. If every woman gets a "Pap" smear on a six-month or yearly basis during this time it is almost certain that cancer will be discovered before it leads to significant vaginal bleeding. In a woman who has gone through menopause, vaginal bleeding is a very strong sign of cancer of the womb or cervix. *Any woman who develops vaginal bleeding after menopause should see a doctor immediately*. Of course an inflammation or tumor of the vaginal wall can cause vaginal bleeding, too, but this is very unusual.

Women who have recently delivered a baby may have vaginal bleeding from retained placenta (afterbirth). Vaginal bleeding during pregnancy may be due to early separation of the placenta or placenta previa (afterbirth situated at the mouth of the womb) and may signify an impending abortion. Therefore *any women with vaginal bleeding during pregnancy should see her doctor immediately*.

What can I do about vaginal bleeding?

Don't just buy more Kotex! Abnormal vaginal bleeding means you should *consult your doctor*. Usually he can determine over the phone whether this is serious enough to require immediate investigation. If he does then he will want to do an immediate "Pap" smear and possibly admit you for a dilatation and curettage (page 307) and do some hormonal and blood studies on you.

What will happen if I don't do anything about it?

If you don't do anything about it the chances are it will clear up on its own. However, any woman who is beyond the menopause is only fooling herself if she does not consult a physician immediately. One more thing: vaginal bleeding does *not* signify that a woman has venereal disease.

Vaginal Discharge

What is a vaginal discharge?

A vaginal discharge is the excessive secretion of a whitish, yellowish, or greenish mucus from the vagina. Every woman has a vaginal discharge normally. However, this is rarely more than enough to cause a couple of spots on her panties each day. It is usually white in color. If the vaginal secretion changes to yellow or green or becomes more profuse, then disease is likely and you should consult your physician. A vaginal discharge is probably one of the most common gynecological problems in women today.

What is the cause of a vaginal discharge?

There are a variety of causes of a vaginal discharge. Pregnancy, for example, may cause an increase in the secretions in the vagina, but this is usually a whitish material. The other common causes of a vaginal discharge are bacteria, particularly gonorrhea, moniliasis (a fungus), Trichomonas (a parasite), and finally a chronic inflammation of the cervix, called cervicitis.

What can I do about a vaginal discharge?

Report to your physician immediately if you ever discover that your normal secretion has changed in color to yellow or green or that it has become more profuse. He will examine you, take smears of your vaginal fluid, stain them and culture them to determine which of the causes or conditions you have. There are many all-purpose vaginal suppositories that will kill whatever fungus, bacteria or parasite is causing the discharge in most cases. However, by the smears and cultures your doctor can determine which type of vaginal infection you have and then give you the most appropriate treatment. Moniliasis vaginitis, which is very common, is treated with Sporastacin cream or nystatin suppositories. Trichamonas parasites are destroyed by Flagyl taken by mouth twice a day. Frequently the husband must be treated also. Gonorrhea is treated with penicillin. It is important to clear up any associated cervicitis in any of these types of infection. I also check on the vaginal hygiene of each patient. Chronic cervicitis can be cured by cauterization, which sometimes requires the patient to be hospitalized.

Is vaginal discharge dangerous?

No.

What will happen if I don't do anything about it?

Nothing will happen as a rule. However, if it is due to gonorrhea, then your child will be affected by it if you become pregnant. Many women automatically think they have a venereal disease when they have a vaginal discharge. They are ashamed to see a doctor. Moreover they may blame their husbands for the infection. Actually moniliasis and Trichimonas are the most common causes of vaginal infection, and they are not venereal diseases.

COMMON DISEASES

Acne

What is acne?

Acne is an inflammation of the skin, sebaceous glands ("oil glands"), and hair follicles, usually involving the face, although it may involve the neck, back, and chest as well.

What is the cause of acne?

The exact cause of acne is not definitely known, but certainly the formation of too much keratin at the mouths of the sebaceous glands and hair follicles is a very important factor. The keratin is the thick yellowish crust formed by the skin to protect us from bacteria and other environmental agents. When the hair follicles and sebaceous glands are blocked, bacteria multiply behind the blockage and the sebaceous material accumulates. This produces severe inflammation. If the multiplication of bacteria is allowed to go on a boil will be produced and a scar will be left by the opening and drainage of the boil.

What are the symptoms and signs of acne?

The primary symptom of acne is a rash of the face, usually a pimply rash, and there may be opening and drainage of the sebaceous glands with pus. As stated above acne may occur on the skin of the back and chest and the same kind of pimply rash will occur there. There is usually no fever or other constitutional symptoms. When acne has progressed for several years there may be scars on the face and some other disfigurements.

What can I do about it?

Your diet is important. You should avoid chocolate, nuts, fried foods, fats, iodized salt, shell fish, cheese and ice cream, and limit your milk ingestion. Personal hygiene is also important. Do not wash your face more than once a day and then scrub it fairly well but not severely. Use a bland soap such as Safeguard. Some patients should wash their faces only with ten percent alcohol. This avoids blockage of the pores by soap. I also advise taking vitamin A every day. There are several useful creams available that your physician will prescribe to dissolve the blackheads and keratin crust. Above all do not squeeze the blackheads or the crusts from the sebaceous glands. When you feel that one of your sores has become infected you must contact your physician so that he can give you an appropriate antibiotic. Doctors have begun prescribing some antibiotics on a regular basis with good results. These include the tetracyclines and erythromycins. Estrogen hormones have been prescribed in some cases with good results as well. X-ray therapy and ultraviolet therapy are reserved for the more resistant cases. Finally, surgery in the form of dermabrasion and chemosurgery may be necessary if your face becomes scarred and disfigured.

Is it dangerous?

No. Acne is not dangerous unless one of your pimples becomes infected to the point that the infection spreads into your system. This is very rare, fortunately.

What can I do to prevent it?

Avoiding rich diets and washing carefully daily but not too frequently is about the only thing I know of to prevent acne.

Alcoholism

What is alcoholism?

Alcoholism is addiction to alcohol. This may be physiological (body dependence) or psychological (emotional dependence) or both. There are probably nine million alcoholics in the United States. Most severe alcoholics consume more than a pint of whiskey or two to three quarts of beer a day. Addiction to wine and whiskey is more common than addiction to beer.

What causes it?

The main cause of alcoholism is psychological, and most patients have a chronic anxiety, hostility or depression. Very few alcoholics are schizophrenic. Alcoholics as a group have a great deal of difficulty expressing anger and often have a lot of subconscious guilt. The more one turns to alcohol to achieve a sense of well-being, the more alcohol he must consume to achieve that state. Eventually a metabolic and physical dependency on alcohol occurs, and the subject develops the shakes, irritability, and confusion if he doesn't have a drink to start the day.

What are the symptoms and signs of it?

Chronic alcoholics usually appear normal except for the smell of alcohol on their breath. They do not stagger or exhibit slurred speech. Their faces are usually ruddy and the voice is husky. The diagnosis of chronic alcoholism is best made during withdrawal. Then there will be shaking of the hands, lips and voice, confusion, sometimes hallucinations, and even convulsions. This condition is called DT's, or delerium tremens. Many patients admit to excessive drinking, but most won't unless they are under pressure.

What can I do about alcoholism?

Admitting to excessive drinking is half the battle. See your physician. He will often refer you for psychiatric help. It is best to be admitted to a hospital alcoholic unit to dry out, but if none is available any hospital bed will do. Tranquilizers, anticonvulsants, vitamins and a special diet are prescribed. It is most important that you vow not to touch a drink again. Joining the local chapter of Alcoholics Anonymous is extremly helpful. The rehabilitation of an alcoholic is often a long and tedious process. We should never give up in despair even though the patient may return to drinking several times before he is finally "on the wagon" for good.

Is it dangerous?

Yes. Alcohol destroys brain cells by the thousands. The brain of an alcoholic is often shrunken and "moth-eaten." The liver is also destroyed. At first it becomes swollen and later shriveled up. The lining of the stomach may also become thinned out and ulcerated. There may be a severe anemia. The pancreas may become inflamed periodically. Anyone of these above conditions may kill the alcoholic. On top of that he is extremely accident prone. It is estimated that in eighty percent of auto accidents one or the other of the drivers was drinking.

What can I do to prevent it?

Eat a well-balanced diet with plenty of vitamins. When you suffer from anxiety or depression get to a doctor for psychotherapy and tranquilizers before you turn to drinking for relief. At the first sign that you need a drink early in the day to "settle your nerves," get professional help.

Appendicitis

What is appendicitis?

Appendicitis is an inflammation of the appendix, a small finger-like projection from the right side of the large bowel. This is the most common surgical emergency of the abdomen.

What is the cause of appendicitis?

Appendicitis may be caused by obstruction of the lumen (the space inside) of the appendix or by infection. Most commonly both factors are involved. The small lumen of the appendix may be obstructed by a fecalith, which is a hard piece of stool, by pinworms, and occasionally by enlargement of the lymph nodes around the mouth of the appendix. If obstruction has occurred then the bacteria that are normally present in the appendix begin to multiply. Occasionally the appendix may be infected by bacteria—often streptococci—that reach it through the blood stream.

What are the symptoms and signs of appendicitis?

At the onset of appendicitis there is usually generalized abdominal pain, but this may become localized to the right lower portion of the abdomen. The pain is not as severe as in gall bladder disease and it is not usually associated with nausea and vomiting. There may or may not be a slight temperature, from 100° to 101°. Pain in the back and down the leg is unusual but can occur. There is usually no diarrhea. Some people who have mild chronic appendicitis may have only moderate abdominal pain periodically without nausea and vomiting, but they do have a poor appetite. Chronic appendicitis was once thought not to exist but now we know better.

What can I do about appendicitis?

If you have abdominal pain that begins around the navel and eventually goes to the lower right area of the abdomen, without severe nausea or vomiting or diarrhea, you should see your doctor for evaluation for possible appendicitis. After he examines you he will probably order a white blood count and a urine test and have a surgeon look at you, too. If the diagnosis is appendicitis the next step is almost invariably surgery. Surgery for appendicitis takes only about twenty to forty-five minutes. Following surgery you will almost immediately feel excellent. You will be out of the hospital within five to seven days. Some physicians do treat appendicitis with antibiotics, but this is not considered the best method with today's remarkable surgery.

What will happen if I don't do anything about it?

Well, occasionally your appendicitis will clear up without any complications, but the usual course is that the appendix ruptures and causes severe peritonitis (infection of your entire abdomen), in which case you will die in fever and prostration, unless you can be helped by antibiotics. Therefore it is a dangerous condition and should not be left untreated.

How can I prevent it?

Prevention of appendicitis is almost impossible. You should take measures to keep from getting pinworms, and treat pinworms as soon as they are noticed, because pinworms may obstruct the lumen in the appendix and cause appendicitis. Pinworms can be prevented by washing your hands before you eat anything and after playing with pets. They can be treated with a single dose of Povan. One sure prevention of appendicitis: if a surgeon operates on you for something else in the abdomen, let him take the appendix out before it causes trouble.

Arthritis and Rheumatism

What are arthritis and rheumatism?

Most lay people call any recurrent ache or pain in their body rheumatism, whether the ache or pain is in the joints, muscles, tendons, or ligaments. However, when one speaks specifically of a joint inflammation one means arthritis.

What causes arthritis?

This can be caused by a variety of etiological agents. The most common form is rheumatoid arthritis, which is a non-specific inflammation of the joints. Another type of arthritis is gout, which is well known to the lay people. In this condition deposits of a crystal called uric acid accumulate in the joints and create irritation. Still another common type is osteoarthritis, which is usually due to degeneration of cartilage and overgrowth of bone around the joints because of continuous use and trauma to the joints. Whether osteoarthritis is due to aging is not clear, but it seems to be definitely related to use of a joint and occurs most frequently in weight-bearing joints. Heredity may play a very important role in osteoarthritis. These are the three major types of arthritis that one sees from day to day. However, rheumatic fever (see page 227) can produce inflammation of the joints, as is well known to many of you. This usually occurs in younger people and may be associated with inflammation of the heart and skin. Also, specific diseases such as streptococcus or tuberculosis may cause joint infections, but these are very rare. It is said that over ten million people in this country suffer from arthritis. While this may be true I would caution the reader not to jump to the conclusion that there are ten million cripples in this country. Only a very small percentage probably less than one hundred thousand, of the people who suffer from a form of arthritis are in any way crippled by it. The people who make up statistics such as this may well include all types of aches and pains in this estimate. I have heard statistics that there are four million or more diabetics, several million epileptics, and several million people with heart conditions. If all the statistics on illnesses are true then it is a wonder that there is anyone out walking the street!

GOUTY ARTHRITIS

What causes gouty arthritis?

The accumulation of uric acid in the body is responsible. This may be from increased production or decreased excretion. There may be increased uric acid production in certain blood diseases, cancer and hereditary diseases. There may be decreased excretion in kidney diseases.

What are the symptoms and signs?

The symptoms of gout are usually swelling, pain, and redness of the proximal (closest to the point of attachment) portion of the big toe. Any joint in the body can be affected by gout, just as in the other forms of arthritis. The pain is so severe that even if the bedclothes touch the affected joint the patient experiences a lot of pain. Although it may occur, there is rarely any fever associated with gout. Patients who have gout sometimes have kidney stones as well. Less frequently gout may involve the bursa (sacs between tendons and bones) or the tendons or ligaments, as it does in rheumatoid arthritis.

What can I do about gout?

For thousands of years a drug has been available called colchicine, which is extremely useful in the acute attack of gout. Aspirin is also effective in the treatment of gout as is cortisone, which does not have to be used on such a long-term basis as it does with rheumatoid arthritis to get permanent relief. Once the patient gets relief from any one of these three drugs there is a drug available called Benemid (probenicid) to lower the uric acid in the person's system. This will help prevent attacks of gout. More recently a drug called allopurinol has been devised that will inhibit the body from forming uric acid; this drug is very effective in preventing attacks of gout, although it does nothing for treating the acute condition. Refraining from exposure to cold, getting adequate exercise, and going on a low purine or uric-acid diet are all helpful in preventing attacks of gout.

What will happen if I do nothing about gout?

Gout is another type of arthritis that is rarely crippling; however, I have seen one or two crippling cases in my practice. The acute attack will gradually subside with bed rest and no other treatment. Very few people die from gout.

Is it dangerous?

I do not consider the vast majority of cases of gout dangerous to the individual.

OSTEOARTHRITIS

What causes osteoarthritis?

We don't know.

What are the symptoms and signs of osteoarthritis?

Osteoarthritis begins with painful swelling and sometimes bony projections over certain joints, particularly the fingers, the knees and toes. Although it is less likely, occasionally a patient experiences fever or an acute red-hot joint swelling secondary to osteoarthritis. X-rays of the joint often reveal evidence of the bony overgrowth around the joint and thinning of the cartilage.

What can I do about osteoarthritis?

In most cases very little needs to be done, but when a joint becomes acutely swollen and painful a local injection of cortisone is an extremely valuable method of treatment. Here again aspirin is useful but it is not quite as effective as it is in rheumatoid arthritis. Patients who are obese could do well to lose weight, as this will improve the arthritis in the weight-bearing joints. Good exercise and physiotherapy are often helpful. If nothing at all is done about osteoarthritis it rarely will develop into a crippling illness. In many cases it will clear up spontaneously without any medical care.

How can I prevent myself from getting this?

There is no known way that this can be done.

RHEUMATOID ARTHRITIS

What causes rheumatoid arthritis?

The cause of rheumatoid arthritis is unknown. Many research investigators have tried to ascribe it to an infection but none of the findings has been well substantiated. The most strongly held theory is that it is caused by a peculiar antibody that develops in the body and actually attacks our own tissues, specifically the joint tissues. (As you probably know, antibodies are usually formed to attack some invading organism, such as a bacteria or virus.) As for influencing factors on arthritis, it seems that emotional illness is extremely important in rheumatoid arthritis.

What are the symptoms and signs of rheumatoid arthritis?

Rheumatoid arthritis usually has its onset with pain, redness, and swelling in any one of the joints but particularly the fingers, knees, or elbows. It may also start with an inflammation of the muscle or ligaments before it actually involves the joints. It may or may not be associated with fever or chills. Sometimes there is weight loss and loss of appetite. Unlike rheumatic fever, rheumatoid arthritis has not been found to follow any specific infections, such as streptococcus, etc.

What can I do about rheumatoid arthritis?

There are many excellent methods of treatment for rheumatoid arthritis today but the most important is aspirin. The aspirin, however, must be taken in the proper dosages (up to three or four tablets four times a day) and for the desired period of time in order to eliminate the inflammation. Some of you may have heard that toxic effects result from a lot of aspirin. These effects are very very infrequent. The most common one is gastritis, or inflammation of the stomach leading to ulcers. If the administration of aspirin is under proper supervision this should be a rare occurrence. I would discourage patients from simply using one or two aspirins when the inflammation develops. If there is a significant amount of inflammation in the joints the aspirin must be taken at least two to three weeks.

Other drugs have been developed that in some cases seem

to be more effective than aspirin. For the past twenty years doctors have tried cortisone or its analogues on their patients with rheumatoid arthritis, with variable degrees of success. Cortisone given orally gives immediate relief but the problem is that as soon as the drug is withdrawn the patient starts up with the same symptoms again. I have refrained from prescribing cortisone over a long period of time because of the dangerous side effects. Cortisone, like aspirin, may lead to ulcers, but it can also lead to hypertension or sugar diabetes, make one more vulnerable to infection, and cause deterioration of the bones in the body. Probably less significant are the emotional disturbances it may cause. Most of all it reduces the body's own ability to form cortisone and after long use of cortisone one may become dependent on it. Cortisone given for short periods or injected locally into the joint is very useful.

Another successful treatment that has been available for a long time is gold treatment, but here again there are many side effects. Only a certain select group of people can get any value from it. These people must be determined by the individual physician.

As a patient you can do most by getting adequate rest and systematic exercising of the joints involved. Your doctor may decide that you need to be hospitalized for a certain period of time for both rest and physiotherapy (in the form of paraffin baths or heat treatment, etc.). Some joints seem to be extremely responsive to cortisone locally. This is less likely to cause systemic complications than is oral cortisone medication. If aspirin is unsuccessful your doctor may try Indocin, which is another new drug, or other drugs at his discretion.

Is rheumatoid arthritis dangerous?

I think this is easily answered by the very few people that are crippled by this disease. Unfortunately, the various foundations that are trying to raise money for research in this disease make it sound as if many people are crippled with this disease. Actually very few are. In the entire time I have been practicing I have seen only four or five people with the crippling form of this disease. In many cases if nothing is done at all the disease may burn itself out in two to five years and leave only a few scars or deformities. However it is more likely that you will have a more favorable prognosis if you get supervision by your physician.

Asthma

What is asthma?

Asthma, in a sense that most lay people understand it, is an allergic condition affecting the lungs that makes people wheeze and get short of breath. Asthma may also be due to other causes and therefore should not be classified as just an allergic disease. You can have cardiac asthma, which is due to the backing up of blood from the heart in a patient with heart failure and which causes congestion of the lungs, and you can have an infectious asthma in which the smaller passages of the lungs are affected by an infection, either bacterial or viral. The symptoms of asthma can be produced also by a foreign body in the lungs such as a peanut. But most cases of asthma are due to an allergy to something, whether it be house dust or mold or some pollen in the air. Asthma is a very common condition and at least forty percent of people who have hay fever actually develop asthma.

What are the symptoms and signs of asthma?

During an asthmatic attack a patient experiences wheezing, in other words his breathing is labored and he makes a lot of noise, sometimes musical, sometimes rasping.

He coughs and has a great deal of difficulty catching his breath. The cough is usually dry but may be productive. The patient breathes rapidly. His pulse may become rapid, although he may not notice this. His chest may also expand because he is unable to expire all the air in it. There is usually no pain in the chest when the patient has asthma. The patient may sneeze frequently and have a runny nose. There is not usually a temperature or a chill with the asthmatic attack, but if the attack gets really severe these could develop.

What can I do about asthma?

Fortunately there are numerous methods of treating asthma, all of which work. The asthmatic attack can be ended abruptly with a shot of adrenalin (extract from the adrenal gland), and this is the usual way it is treated in emergency rooms. In addition the patient receives oxygen so that each breath can be more effective with a greater amount of oxygen in it. A substance similar to adrenalin may be put into an inhaler and in this way sucked or blown into the respiratory passages through the nose or mouth. In the severe attack the patient may need a shot of cortisone or cortisone preparation. Some attacks end spontaneously within two to three minutes but the majority may last several hours if not treated in the manner described above. Other drugs, such as aminophylline, a derivative of caffeine or tranquilizers may also be needed to stop the attack. In more severe attacks the patient will have to be admitted to the hospital and sometimes a tracheotomy must be performed, but this is very unusual and I would caution the asthmatic reading this article not to be alarmed about this possibility. Of course, for those asthmatics who have associated pneumonia or other infections in the lungs, antibiotics are given. Expectorants are also of great value in treating the asthmatic.

For the prevention of chronic asthmatic attacks it is necessary to get desensitized for the particular allergy causing the attacks. For instance, if you are allergic to house mold then you will get shots weekly from your doctor containing the particular house mold causing your condition. This is called desensitization. Those people whose attacks are precipitated by emotional causes are given tranquilizers and sometimes psychotherapy. Another excellent preventative is to have an electronic filter system in your house, either attached to your furnace or in the form of a portable unit that you can carry from room to room, particularly if you are allergic to house dust or molds. The doctor also should study you with a chest x-ray, pulmonary function tests, and other tests to make sure you don't have any other condition such as heart failure or tuberculosis.

Is asthma dangerous?

Asthma can be dangerous in a small percentage of cases if it is allowed to continue without treatment but as I said before many attacks end by themselves. It becomes obvious that it is dangerous when the patient gets blue and delirious and even comatose. Then treatment is life-saving.

What will happen if I don't do anything about asthma?

The complications of asthma are heart failure and, of course, severe coma and death during the acute stage. If you have chronic recurring attacks you may live a long life having only these attacks. They may eventually disappear by themselves. However, with recurrent attacks eventually the patient may develop pulmonary emphysema, which as you may know is sometimes fatal. In emphysema the lung passages are dilated and obstructed; it is usually an irreversible obstruction because there is also fibrosis of the passages. The bronchi become chronically infected. At all times the lung contains more air than it should and, worst of all, that air is locked in.

How can I prevent myself from having asthmatic attacks?

As I said above the best prevention for asthmatic attacks is to see your doctor and find out the cause of your asthma. If it is determined that it is due to an allergen then it is wise to get desensitization for this particular allergen by weekly shots from your doctor. It is also wise to have your own adrenalin on hand. The doctor will teach you how to administer it during an attack. There are some pills that can be taken during an attack that if placed under the tongue work almost as effectively as the shot. Aside from desensitization with the allergens you should not expose yourself to cold. You should avoid anything that would cause severe emotional excitement. Never overexert yourself physically. Avoid irritants such as tobacco and toxic fumes.

Boils

What are boils?

Boils are little infections of the hair follicles or the sebaceous glands adjacent to the hair follicle. This infection is usually caused by staphylococcus bacteria that multiply in the follicle canal or in the sebaceous gland. Occasionally the infection may be so severe that the sebaceous gland ruptures and the infection extends into the skin around the follicle as well. There are other organisms that can cause boils but it is usually staphylococcus. I feel that the majority of boils is due to either lack of washing in the area or too much washing. If the skin is washed too often then the natural bacteria and oils are taken away and this makes it easier for enemy bacteria to invade. Of course if the person's general nutrition and general physical condition are bad it is easier for these organisms to invade the skin and hair follicles also.

The signs of a boil are swelling, redness, and pus exuding from the hair follicle. Not every red lump in the skin is a boil. A lump in the skin may also be due to a streptococcal cellulitis or infection of the bone underneath the skin, among other things.

What can I do about a boil?

A boil is usually treated by soaking and then opening and draining with a knife. An antibiotic is usually given by mouth, preferably one of the new penicillins that is more specific for staphylococcus. It is important that you take the antibiotic for the prescribed length of time, because if it is given for only a short length of time the infection may flare up again. You may need a surgeon to open and drain the boils, particularly when they are large, since they may extend into the surrounding skin and blood and cause a blood infection that could result in death. People who have frequent boils in various parts of the body should consider their own personal hygiene, particularly whether they are washing too frequently or not often enough. It may also be that staphylococcus is circulating in their blood, not in amounts sufficient to cause any major symptoms, and is being transferred from one boil to another or one hair follicle to another through the body by way of the blood stream. In this case an antibiotic must be taken over a long period of time to eradicate the organism.

Bursitis

What is bursitis?

Bursitis is an inflammation of the bursa—a fluid-containing sac between a tendon or muscle and a bone. This inflammation, which is not usually caused by bacteria or a virus, is due to deposits of calcium in the tendons or muscle underneath the bursa. Bursitis may occur anywhere in the body, but the most commonly known place for it to occur is in the shoulder. It can also occur in the elbow at the ulnar bursa or at the radial or the ulnar joint, where it is called tennis elbow. It can occur in the bursae about the knee or the hip. As is well known this is a very common affliction. It probably affects ten percent of adults at one time or another, although most do not seek treatment for this.

What are the signs or symptoms of bursitis?

The most common sign of bursitis is pain in the area of the affected bursa. Of course since it is most often the shoulder bursa, this is the most likely place for pain. The pain is usually excruciating in the acute stage, but in the chronic type of bursitis it may be mild. With the pain there is usually limitation of motion of the joint. Sometimes in bursitis of the shoulder you cannot raise your arm above the horizontal. In a rare case, the shoulder can be almost frozen. In addition there may be swelling or increase in temperature over the affected area, but there is rarely any fever or chills. Bursitis is not produced by a bacteria or virus. On examination there may be swelling noted, as well as crepitus (crackling in the joints).

What can I do about it?

The best treatment for acute bursitis is an injection of cortisone with a little Novacain. Sometimes two to three injections may be necessary before the pain subsides. In addition, cortisone or aspirin may be given by mouth, and the doctor will probably prescribe something such as Darvon or even codeine for pain. It is important to keep the arm at rest during the initial stage of the treatment (forty-eight to seventy-two hours). Therefore a sling is often prescribed.

Is it dangerous?

No! You will not die of it. However, if it becomes chronic it may freeze the joint involved and cause disability.

What can I do to prevent it?

Unfortunately, very little. Overuse of any joint in the body may contribute to bursitis there, but few people can avoid this. Limiting calcium intake will not help.

Cancer

What is cancer?

Cancer is the rapid independent multiplication of a cell or group of cells in the body. Cancers are often referred to as tumors. Cancers may originate in any organ. Some organs seem to be more likely to have cancers than others. All cancers are considered *malignant;* that is, that they may spread from one organ to another once they have dug into the particular organ that they originate from. Cancers may spread through the blood, the lymph glands, or by direct extension. When a patient mentions that he has a tumor he may or may not mean that he has cancer. Some tumors are *benign;* that is, that they do not spread from one organ to another, although they may cause pressure on another organ because of its close proximity.

What is the cause of cancer?

No known cause of cancer has been found to this date. It is speculated that some small virus or nucleoprotein may be responsible for most cancers. Leukemia in chickens has been found to be due to a virus. It has been found that certain chemicals in cigarettes predispose to cancers in various organs. Everyone is anxiously awaiting for the cause of cancer to be found.

What are the symptoms and signs of cancer?

The symptoms and signs of cancer will vary according to the organ in which the cancer originates. Certain general statements can be made however. Most patients with cancer lose weight. Often they lose their appetite and feel weak. Often there will be bleeding from the organ where the cancer is growing. Thus if there is a cancer of the lung a person may cough up blood; if there is cancer of the stomach a patient may vomit blood; and if there is cancer of the rectum the patient may pass blood in the stool. Beyond this the most common symptom of cancer is a lump in the body. The lump may be in the breast, in the abdomen, on the skin, or anywhere in the body. It may be in the testicles or the lymph glands. Cancer in women occurs most commonly in the breast and next most commonly in the womb, the mouth of the womb, the ovaries, and finally in the lower intestinal tract and rectum. Cancer in men is most common in the lung; it is next most common in the intestinal tract and third most common in the prostate gland. It is wise to discuss the symptoms of each of these kinds of cancer because they are so common.

In cancer of the breast there is usually a lump discovered. This is usually painless. This lump often causes some deformity of the breast involved and there may be a lump under the armpit as well. There may be a discharge of blood or mucus from the nipple. Cancer of the womb or the mouth of the womb usually causes abnormal vaginal bleeding in between periods or else a large amount of bleeding at the time of the period. In addition there may be bleeding after intercourse. However cancer of the mouth of the womb (cervix) usually does not cause these symptoms until it is well advanced.

Cancer of the intestinal tract usually causes vomiting of blood or blood in the stools. This may cause a black stool or the stool may be bright red, depending on the part of the intestinal tract involved. There may also be anemia, loss of weight, loss of appetite, diarrhea or constipation. In cancer of the lung there is a rapid loss of weight, loss of appetite, weakness, occasionally fever, occasional pneumonia and most frequently coughing up of blood or mucus. The cough may be dry, however.

Finally, in cancer of the prostate there is occasionally obstruction to the flow of urine, the urinary stream becomes weak and there is dribbling and difficulty initiating urination.

Any one of these cancers may become apparent by metastasis (spread) to another organ. For example, a cancer of the breast may first be discovered when a patient comes to the doctor complaining of pain in her bones and on examination he finds a lump in the bone. A cancer of the lung may be first discovered by an enlarged liver.

What can I do about cancer?

The most important thing to do about cancer is to prevent it. Everyone should stop smoking. There should be a tremendous campaign against environmental pollution. Don't take drugs unless you have to. There are other things that could be suggested for individual cancers. More important than this is a frequent checkup by your family physician. Report to your family physician any time that you have significant weight loss, the passage of blood from any organ system, loss of appetite or persistent fever. When you first discover any sign of possible cancer, report to your doctor immediately. In most cases he will advise surgery. This surgery can be limited to the organ involved or it may be extensive with the removal of the lymph glands near the organ; sometimes he will suggest the removal of the metastasized portion of the tumor when it has spread to another organ. Some tumors can be treated by radiation alone, but radiation is most commonly applied in conjunction with surgery. In addition there are numerous drugs that can be used to fight cancer once it has spread from the site of origin. These are called chemotherapy agents. They are most useful in therapy of cancer of the blood such as leukemia or Hodgkin's disease.

Is cancer dangerous?

The answer to this is obvious. Cancer is a dangerous disease and unless it is discovered early it means almost certain death. However because of frequent "Pap" smears, cancer of the cervix in women has been detected early. Also because women examine their own breasts and get frequent breast examinations by their family physicians the number of deaths from breast cancer has been cut down considerably. Finally frequent chest x-rays have helped save a few cases of cancer of the lung, notably Arthur Godfrey and other stars. Frequent proctoscopic examinations have prevented many deaths and many cases of disability from cancer of the rectum and sigmoid. Cancer of the stomach, lungs and many organs remain ninety to ninety-five percent fatal.

What can I do to prevent cancer?

As mentioned above the most important treatment of cancer is prevention. That is why physicians advise patients to stop smoking, to see their physicians for physical examinations, and have "Pap" smears for women and many other blood tests to find cancer early. Beyond this, eating meals regularly, proper sleep, rest and exercise and avoiding environmental pollutants may prevent cancer!

Cataracts

What are cataracts?

A cataract is not an expensive car! It is a clouding or opacification of the lens of the eye. This is usually a gradual process, taking a few years before sight is impaired. However, some children are born with cataracts (called congenital).

What causes them?

Cataracts may be congenital (present at birth), in which case they are hereditary or caused by some disease the mother had while carrying the baby, such as German measles. Cataracts occurring during later years may be due to aging or diabetes mellitus (page 144).

What can I do about them?

Most cataracts are easily removed surgically. However, if only one eye is affected or if your vision is fairly good, your ophthalmologist will probably delay surgery. Do not be impatient with him. The surgery is not without occasional complications and so a "bird in the hand is worth two in the bush." Regular checkups by your ophthalmologist are your best bet. Cataracts cannot be dissolved by medicine.

What will happen if I don't do anything about them?

Obviously you will eventually lose your sight, but this may take several years. In any case, cataracts are not life-threatening.

How can I prevent them?

By getting regular checkups for diabetes and cataracts that result from aging. They cannot be prevented yet. Women carrying a child should avoid German measles, smoking and drugs of any kind.

Colitis

What is colitis?

Colitis is an inflammation of the colon. The most common forms of this are spastic colitis and ulcerative colitis. In spastic colitis there are recurrent spasms of the intestines and the secretion of large amounts of mucus, which is jammed up into the large intestine. There are no ulcerations of the lining of the intestines as a rule. In ulcerative colitis, however, the entire large bowel or colon has chronic inflammation and ulceration. In this disease there is also a large amount of mucus secreted. There is also bleeding from the ulcerations.

What causes colitis?

The cause of spastic colitis is unknown, but most often these people are extremely nervous and tense. The cause of ulcerative colitis is also unknown. This has been variously ascribed to allergies and hypersensitivity. There seems to be a hereditary trend. It may also be brought on by anxiety or suppressed hostility or depression. Other forms of colitis may be due to bacteria or a parasite, as in amebic colitis. Diverticulitis, discussed elsewhere, may cause a type of colitis.

What are the symptoms and signs of colitis?

In ulcerative colitis there is persistent diarrhea, often ten to thirty times a day, accompanied by severe cramps. There is often large amounts of mucus and blood associated with the diarrhea. Those of you who have had moderate gastroenteritis are familiar with severe diarrhea that occurs for two or three days, but if this diarrhea should persist then one must consult his physician to rule out ulcerative colitis, amebic colitis or spastic colitis. In spastic colitis, however, there is often diarrhea alternating with constipation. In fact some of these patients may not have diarrhea at all but only constipation. The stool is rarely bloody, but there may be large amounts of mucus as in ulcerative colitis. In ulcerative colitis the patient may often have fever or appear acutely ill and toxic, but in mucus, or spastic, colitis there are rarely any constitutional manifestations.

What can I do about colitis?

The most important thing to do is to consult your physician so that he can have x-rays in the form of a barium enema performed to find out if you have ulcerative colitis. And he will also perform a sigmoidoscopy to see if he can actually visualize the ulcerations in your bowel. Then he will put you on a proper diet, a bowel relaxant, and maybe a sulfa drug to try to eliminate any overgrowth of bacteria in your intestine. Occasionally he will have to use cortisone if you have ulcerative colitis. When ulcerative colitis has persisted for years and has gotten continuously worse or there has been an acute toxic attack with shock or other constitutional symptoms, then a surgeon must be called in to remove your large bowel.

Is it dangerous?

Mucus colitis, or spastic colitis, is not a dangerous condition. A person requires little treatment if he desires to save money. Ulcerative colitis if not taken care of will result in rupture of the bowels and sometimes severe abscess formation and shock, and it can lead to death. In addition, patients with ulcerative colitis may develop cancer if they do not take care of themselves.

What will happen if I don't do anything about it?

With mucus colitis if you don't do anything about it very little will happen. With ulcerative colitis if you don't do anything about it you may develop complications such as perforation of the bowel, abscess formation, constriction of the bowel, or shock.

The Common Cold

What is the common cold?

The common cold is an infection of the upper respiratory passages.

What causes the common cold?

The common cold is not just one infection; it is many. It can be caused by various viruses. It is rarely caused by bacteria. The common cold can usually be defined as an inflammation of the nasal passages and its related areas, such as sinuses and the eustachian canal (the canal that leads from the nose to the ears), and the throat, trachea and larynx.

The common cold rarely affects the lungs or the bronchial passages, but a few viruses can attack this area. Of course many of the viruses are the Coxsackie variety. Another one is the virus of pharyngoconjunctival fever which may affect the conjunctiva of the eyes. Some patients who have what is considered a common cold may have viral influenza.

What are the symptoms and signs of a common cold?

The symptoms of a common cold are usually a runny nose, headache, postnasal drip, sore throat, occasionally earache, and frequently a cough that is usually dry in character. In addition one may experience systemic symptoms of slight nausea, slight fever, generalized fatigue, and occasionally muscular aches and pains.

Is it dangerous?

Generally, no! For the average person in a population of fairly good health this is not a dangerous illness. If nothing is done about it, it will probably clear up by itself. The reason the common cold is so common is because very few people develop a prolonged immunity to the viruses that cause colds. The only way to prevent it would be to avoid exposure to people who have a common cold and to keep your diet fortified with vitamins and the basic seven ingredients in a good diet.

What can I do about it?

Once you have a cold your general care is more important than any specific drug. For instance, one should get plenty of rest, have good humidity in your room, drink a lot of fluids, and not load your stomach with food. Staying indoors is generally a good idea but if one does not expose himself to cold temperatures too long, being outdoors is not necessarily harmful as long as you bundle up well. As for specific medications for the common cold, we have none. Many of my patients ask for a shot of penicillin and they are very sure that this will help. However, generally the antibiotics such as penicillin do nothing for the common cold unless there is a bacterial complication. I usually prescribe aspirin, two to three tablets every four hours, a nasal decongestant such as Dristan, which is commonly bought without a prescription. Our prescription drugs of similar action are Actifed and antihistamines. If the nose is continuously blocked, a nasal spray may be of some help but this should not be used too frequently. Frequent use of a nasal decongestant such as Neo-Synephrine will actually harm the nasal mucosa and make the cold worse.

Where your doctor can be of most help is in treating the complications. The common complications of a cold are sinusitis, which is often due to a bacteria, otitis media (infection of the ear), which is often due to a bacteria, and pneumonia. All three of these complications are best treated with an antibiotic such as penicillin or Terramycin. One shot of penicillin, however, will not cure such complications and one needs to take antibiotics for at least five to eight days. People who are in most danger with the common cold are those who already have a respiratory or cardiac disease, such as heart failure or pulmonary emphysema. Both of these diseases have a tendency to make one susceptible to pneumonia. Also, children and some adults who have chronic ear infections are in more danger when they get a cold because they may get a new ear infection. If you develop one of these complications of a cold then almost invariably you will develop a temperature. If you develop pneumonia your cough will become productive of a yellowish thick mucus material. You may even develop shortness of breath. In summary a common cold is an infection due to viruses that cannot be treated with antibiotics, but its complications frequently require the administration of antibiotics. If you take good care of yourself, drink a lot of fluids and take aspirin you will probably not have to consult your physician.

Concussions and Head Injuries

What are concussions and head injuries?

A concussion is a jarring of the brains causing loss of consciousness or temporary amnesia. Head injuries may include lacerations of the scalp, skull fractures, concussions or intracranial hemorrhage. Concussion and head injuries are frequent occurrences at all ages because of the numerous auto accidents. Thus physicians see these injuries frequently in the emergency rooms.

What causes concussions and head injuries?

The usual cause is a blow to the head; for example, as the patient is thrown forward in an automobile accident. The patient can be said to have a concussion if he receives enough of a blow to make him unconscious. Usually this period of unconsciousness lasts only for five seconds to three minutes but it may last as much as forty-eight hours. When there is a concussion the brain is jarred about and there is often edema or swelling in the brain itself. In more severe concussions there are very minute hemorrhages in various areas of the brain. If these hemorrhages become big they may form a "clot" in the brain. Sometimes the clot may develop just beneath the skull in what we call the extradural space or the subdural space. In these cases the condition is known as extradural (or epidural) hematoma or subdural hematoma respectively. These are the most serious complications of a head injury, as most skull fractures heal very easily and do not cause any symptoms whatsoever. However, if the skull fracture is depressed and pressing on the brain then, of course, symptoms may develop. The serious complications from a head injury or a concussion develop in only one or two percent of head injuries. Therefore it is really foolish to panic when a person passes out after a blow to the head.

What are the symptoms and signs of a head injury and concussion?

The symptoms of a head injury are usually a short period of unconsciousness followed by a headache, dizziness, and often nausea and vomiting if there definitely is a concussion. A person cannot be said definitely to have a concussion, however, unless there was a short period of unconsciousness or there was amnesia for the accident and for some period afterwards. If there was a laceration to the skull during the head injury then there will naturally be bleeding but there may be just subcutaneous bleeding with a bruise of the skull and swelling of the area where the blow occurred. For at least two or three days after the concussion or head injury the victim may experience head pain and nausea. In addition, he may become forgetful and have headaches and dizziness for up to six months or a year. A few patients with a concussion develop epilepsy one to fifteen years after the accident.

What can I do about a concussion or a head injury?

The most important thing is to see your family doctor or go to the emergency room. The doctor will order an x-ray of the skull to make sure there is no fracture. However more important than the x-ray is a thorough examination of the eyes, ears, nose, and throat by the doctor. If the patient has definitely passed out then a twenty-four to forty-eight hour period of observation is necessary to make sure that no extradural or subdural bleeding has occurred to form a clot on the brain. This is usually done in the hospital, but if the mother is an alert person and reliable it can be done at home if she is willing to stay up throughout the night and waken the child frequently. The advantage of being in the hospital is that the blood pressure and pulse can be checked frequently to observe for these complications. A special device has been developed called the echoencephalogram, which can show pretty quickly whether there is a clot developing in the brain. This is a new type of brain-wave test that can be applied frequently during the period of observation of the child or person involved. If a clot is discovered a neurosurgeon must operate to remove the clot.

What will happen if I don't do anything about a head injury?

In most cases you will get away scot-free without complications or any pain afterwards. It is foolish to take this chance and you should see your physician whenever you have any significant blow to the head with a period of unconsciousness.

Contagious Diseases of Childhood

These diseases are grouped together because aside from scarlet fever they are very mild and require no treatment and do not cause any serious complications as a rule.

CHICKEN POX

What causes chicken pox?

Chicken pox is caused by a virus. This virus is a relative probably identical with the virus of herpes zoster, or shingles.

What are the symptoms and signs of chicken pox?

Chicken pox develops with a blister-like rash beginning on the trunk or abdomen and spreading to the face and the arms and legs. The blisters are usually about the size of a bead but may be smaller or larger in various areas of the body. They usually appear in groups. The blisters itch severely, and this is the reason children scratch themselves and cause permanent scarring. There is usually no temperature nor any sore throat or pink eye as there may be in measles. The rash usually disappears in a week but may continue for ten days to two weeks.

What can I do about chicken pox?

Nothing needs to be done because the condition will clear up on its own without treatment. Nobody has ever died from chicken pox to my knowledge. There are no severe complications other than infection of the blisters by bacteria.

Is it dangerous?

No, no one has ever died of chicken pox to my knowledge. There are no serious complications.

What can I do to prevent chicken pox?

The best thing to do is to stay away from a person who has chicken pox. Anybody who has chicken pox should be kept in isolation until the blisters have disappeared.

MEASLES

What causes measles?

Measles is caused by a virus. It may be spread from personal contact by coughing and sneezing. Fortunately the virus that carries measles is destroyed by air and sunlight. Measles is one of the oldest diseases known to man.

What are the symptoms and signs of measles?

A child with measles develops fever and a sore throat, usually inflammation of the eyes, and occasionally coughing and sneezing. Then he develops a rash, usually beginning on the face and spreading over the body from head to toe. The rash is a maculo-papular rash, which means that it is small red pimples with a red circle around them. It usually does not develop into blisters as in chicken pox. The rash is itchy but not nearly as itchy as chicken pox. The rash usually disappears within six to ten days. In contrast to German measles, there is not usually a marked enlargement of the lymph nodes in the neck and behind the ears, and of course the rash lasts longer. If your physician looks inside the mouth he can see little white spots, called Koplik's spots, adjacent to the molars and this helps make a diagnosis.

What can I do about it?

In general there is no need to do anything but rest and stay away from other people. Aspirin is very good for keeping the temperature down; also drink a lot of fluids and don't take heavy meals. An antibiotic would be prescribed only if your doctor felt that you had developed a complication such as pneumonia secondary to the bronchitis of measles.

Is it dangerous?

No. Occasionally a patient with measles may develop an ear infection or an encephalitis, but this is unusual.

What can I do to prevent measles?

The best thing to do is take the measles vaccine, which is now available to all children. It is very cheap and gives almost life-long immunity. The other main precaution is to stay away from people with measles unless you see them in the sunlight outdoors. Your doctor will keep you away from other people if you have measles so that you will not transmit it to other people. A child should not return to school until the rash is gone. This may be as long as ten days from the onset of measles.

GERMAN MEASLES

What causes German measles?

German measles is caused by a virus. It is a very contagious and a very common disease.

What are the symptoms and signs of German measles?

German measles usually begins without much of a temperature but with a swelling in the lymph nodes in the neck and in the back of the ears. This swelling would not usually be noted by the parents. Then a small maculo-papular rash develops on the face and chest and then spreads over the whole body. The rash changes from little macules to papules (pimples) and disappears within three days in most cases. There is rarely any severe temperature with German measles as there is with regular measles. There is very little conjunctivitis or bronchitis with German measles. The rash never becomes pustular or blister-like and therefore does not exude much material, in contrast to chicken pox.

What can I do about German measles?

There is little treatment necessary in German measles because the disease is self-limiting. Aspirin can be given to bring down the temperature and little else is needed. If a pregnant woman or a woman who is possibly pregnant develops German measles or is exposed to it then gamma globulin should be administered immediately. The possibility of a therapeutic abortion must be considered as well, depending on what month of gestation the woman is in.

Is German measles dangerous?

Few if any people die of German measles. However it is dangerous if it occurs in a pregnant woman, because it may inflict severe disease on the infant. The infant may be born with a congenital heart defect or some other unusual distortion of the body.

What can I do to prevent German measles?

A very excellent vaccine for German measles is now developed and is being given to most women before puberty. It is also being given to *un*married adult women who have not had measles and can assure the doctor that they have no possibility of becoming pregnant for a while. Married women who have not had the German measles and desire to get the vaccine can have it if they are put on birth control pills at the same time or refrain from intercourse for a short time. The other way to prevent it is to not be exposed to anyone with German measles.

MUMPS

What is the cause of mumps?

Mumps is a very common contagious disease of childhood caused by a virus. While it is not severe in children, in adult males it can produce a serious consequence.

What are the symptoms and signs of mumps?

It hardly need be mentioned that mumps causes swelling on one or both sides of the face, giving the person a comical appearance. This is because the virus affects the parotid glands, which are salivary glands. The swelling usually pushes the ear out on the side of involvement. The virus may also affect the submaxillary gland, another salivary gland, which would cause enlargement beneath the jaw. There is usually stiffness of the jaw and difficulty swallowing. There is no rash. Temperature is mild if it occurs at all. By looking inside the mouth your physician may discover swelling of the Stensen's duct, which is the duct that leads from the parotid gland to the mouth. This helps him make the diagnosis. Mumps occasionally spreads through the nervous system and causes meningitis; but the most frequent complication of mumps is orchitis, or inflammation of the testicles, in adult males. In this case it may cause sterility and this is why mumps is dangerous.

What can I do about mumps?

There is little treatment necessary. If you stay in bed and stay away from other people, drink lots of fluids and take aspirin for any significant temperature elevation you will have no problems. In an adult male of course the spread to the testicles can cause an awful lot of pain and sometimes hospitalization for treatment with injectable analgesics (pain relievers) may be necessary. Cortisone and A.C.T.H. may be given in cases of orchitis to reduce the swelling of the testicles.

Is it dangerous?

No, mumps is not dangerous. It has rarely killed anybody and the only serious thing that it can do is cause sterility in the adult male.

What can I do to prevent mumps?

There is now a mumps vaccine, which should be taken by adult males who have never had mumps. It is also being given to kids in many cases. Other than that you should stay away from anyone who has been infected with mumps. Children with mumps should be kept at home from school until all visible swelling is gone. This usually takes about two weeks.

SCARLET FEVER

What is the cause of scarlet fever?

Scarlet fever is caused by streptococcal bacteria. These usually infect the tonsils and throat and then they give off a toxin that gets into the blood stream and goes to the skin and causes the goose bumps of scarlet fever. The toxin may also spread to other organs of the body, causing more trouble.

What are the symptoms and signs of scarlet fever?

Scarlet fever is usually ushered in by a sore throat and a high fever, sometimes 102° to 104°. There is often nausea and vomiting and headache. About twenty-four hours after the onset of the fever the rash may develop. This begins about the face and neck and spreads throughout the body. The rash is a goose-bump type of rash and there is erythema, or a beet red appearance to the body. The tongue becomes bright red and sometimes there is swelling of the tissues of the tongue and tiny pits, giving the tongue the semblance of a strawberry. Sometimes there is severe prostration, and there may be disease of the kidneys and other organs.

What can I do about scarlet fever?

Scarlet fever is not dangerous today because a shot or two of penicillin will clear it up without much difficulty. Nevertheless you must take aspirin and lots of fluids, and stay in bed during the initial phase. While this used to be an illness of two to three weeks with six to eight weeks of convalescence, now it is a three-day illness and a child need stay out of school for only three days. Unlike the other contagious diseases of childhood, scarlet fever is caused by bacteria and therefore cured by penicillin.

Is it dangerous?

No. Scarlet fever is no longer a dangerous disease because it can be cured by penicillin before complications develop.

What can I do to prevent it?

Very little can be done to prevent scarlet fever because many people carry the streptococcus in their throat. It is only your own lowered resistance that makes you susceptible to it. The best thing to do is to take a one-a-day vitamin, get a good diet and get plenty of sleep and exercise. For those patients with rheumatic fever, discussed in another chapter, penicillin and sulfonamides have been prescribed on a daily basis to prevent them from getting a strep infection and to prevent scarlet fever.

MISCELLANEOUS

Three other infectious diseases of childhood—whooping cough, diphtheria and poliomyelitis—are rarely seen today. This is because of three excellent vaccines that have been developed for these diseases; most children now get a whooping cough, diphtheria and poliomyelitis vaccine before the age of one year. Smallpox vaccine is also given to children and this has virtually wiped this disease off the map. It therefore seems unnecessary to discuss the symptoms and signs of these four diseases because the prevention has become so effective.

A word of caution: Parents must make sure that their children receive the necessary vaccines for these diseases (see page 322 for discussion of smallpox vaccine), so that dangerous epidemics do not recur. Several children died of polio in a very recent epidemic in Connecticut.

Cuts and Abrasions

What are cuts and abrasions?

A *cut* is a small or large nick made in the skin by a sharp object, either causing separation of the entire skin or just the superficial layers. An *abrasion* is a scraping of the skin leading to many small minute cuts in the skin but without causing complete separation of the skin through the deep layers.

What can I do about cuts and abrasions?

Abrasions may require very little treatment other than cleansing and application of an antiseptic ointment. The use of iodine and other toxic substances is to be discouraged unless there is an extreme amount of dirt in the wound. Iodine may actually destroy the tissue and delay the healing. Superficial cuts can be handled the same way as the abrasions, just by cleansing and applying a Band-Aid. I would not apply iodine to this either. I have found *gentian violet* very useful when applied to abrasions because it is antiseptic and antifungal; it dries the area very nicely so that a scab can be formed.

With deeper cuts you must have a doctor suture them. If you cannot decide whether you have a superficial or a deep cut, then see your physician by all means. I have seen many patients with deep cuts treated without suturing; in such cases it takes from ten days to a month for the healing to take place. In addition infection may set into a deep cut if it is not sutured. When I was a boy it was common for deep cuts to be left unsutured, and I have a couple scars on my body from cuts that were not sutured.

In addition it is very important that you have a booster dose of tetanus toxoid whenever you have a cut or an abrasion with a lot of dirt in it. You do not require a booster shot if you have had one within four years. If you have never received tetanus toxoid then you must have tetanus antitoxin, either the human type or the horse serum.

Diabetes Mellitus

What is diabetes mellitus?

Most laymen probably consider that diabetes is simply too much sugar in the blood or urine. While this is true, most physicians define diabetes as a condition in which there is relatively too little insulin in the body to get rid of the sugar. Today we are even more sophisticated and we realize that diabetes also involves a defect in the ability to metabolize fat and protein as well as carbohydrate. But for the laymen I think that the expression of too much sugar is adequate to explain what diabetes is.

What is the cause of diabetes mellitus?

The cause of diabetes is now considered to be heredity. If you have diabetes, somewhere in your ancestory there was someone who also had diabetes or would have had diabetes if he had lived long enough. It used to be that people blamed diabetes on the fact that a person overate. While it is true that the person prone to develop diabetes will develop it sooner if he is a big eater and becomes fat, he must first have the hereditary characteristics that make him prone to diabetes. In research on diabetes it was discovered that removal of the pancreas in dogs caused diabetes. A few diabetics, of course, owe their illness to the fact that their pancreas was either removed surgically or destroyed by some disease.

What is the incidence of diabetes?

Diabetes has become a great public health problem, since there are four million diabetics in the United States alone. It is the seventh cause of death in the United States. However, this should not frighten you because two-thirds of the cases of diabetes develop in older people. Moreover, it is easily controlled by proper diet and the use of pills. In fact some people can eliminate their elevated blood sugars merely by losing weight. Furthermore, the new insulins are very well synthesized and there are long-acting insulins that are easy to use and don't require so many injections. In general diabetes is not as life-threatening as it used to be.

What are the symptoms of diabetes mellitus?

People used to think a diabetic was someone who was very fat and kept eating a lot of sugar, stuffing his mouth with sweets. Actually, the person who is developing diabetes usually begins to lose weight, becomes thirsty, and eats a great deal but not just sugar. He also goes to the bathroom a lot, since the sugar that has accumulated in his blood passes over to his urine and takes with it a lot of the body water. Therefore he must drink a lot of water to replace this. In medical terms we call these symptoms polyphagia (eating a lot), polydipsia (drinking a lot) and polyuria (urinating a lot), and weight loss.

In addition the diabetic becomes very weak because he cannot use the sugar in his blood for energy in his muscle cells and other cells in his body. Often the diabetic may note a different smell in his urine, which results from the sugar or acetone excreted in his urine. Acetone is a product from the breakdown of fat; and since the diabetic cannot use sugar he must resort to using fat and protein for energy. Since the body often cannot get rid of the breakdown products of fat fast enough, they accumulate in the blood in the form of acetone and other acids called ketones. Since many people are reluctant to complain about symptoms such as these, aside from the weakness, they often do not get to the doctor before coma develops. They may complain more of blurred vision, a boil that fails to heal, a bad rash either in their genitals or in some other area of the body or a kidney infection. Fortunately today we have public health screening programs where sugar is tested frequently. Also doctors are stressing periodical physical examinations that include blood tests for sugar. In addition, routine urine tests are performed frequently. Diabetes can be picked up very early by what we call a two-hour postprandial blood sugar, where blood sugar is drawn two hours after a person has eaten. A normal person can eliminate the sugar from the blood very fast after eating a meal with a lot of sugar in it but the diabetic can't. To discover diabetes is one of the main reasons you should have a physical at least once a year after you reach adulthood, particularly if there is a hereditary history of diabetes.

What can I do about diabetes?

Since the discovery of insulin in 1921 more methods of treating diabetes have been developed that enable the diabetic to live almost a normal life and a normal life span. The vast majority of older diabetics do not require insulin. More important to all diabetics and particularly to those who do not require insulin is the proper diet. It has been found that keeping the diet exactly to the minimum in calories will keep the body's insulin requirements to a minimum; therefore, many diabetics can get along without extra insulin subcutaneously. The contents of the diet will vary with what each doctor feels is most important. One of the most important things is eliminating free sugar from the diet so that the blood sugar will not rise rapidly after a meal. This means that you may have a balance of carbohydrates, fat and protein. In the past diets were given that contained very few carbohydrates for fear that any amount of carbohydrates would elevate the blood sugar too much. Today we believe that the total quantity of the calories in the diet is more important than the quality.

Diabetics who are overweight must reduce to normal. The dietary caloric allowance will be calculated on the basis of their normal weight for their height and build. Many people can "cure" their diabetes simply by losing weight.

After the new diabetic is put on a diet then his urine and blood sugar are tested frequently, particularly if he is young, so that the amount of insulin required can be calculated.

Many older diabetics do not need to take insulin. They can get rid of the high blood sugar by taking a pill that will stimulate the body to produce more insulin or will help utilize the sugar in their body more efficiently.

Various pills that have been used are Orinase, Dymelor, Tolinase, D.B.I. and Diabinese. Recent literature has stated that these are useless and are no more helpful than diet alone. I think that we should have much more information regarding these drugs before we stop using them, particularly since it has not been proven that they are harmful to the body.

When a diabetic has to take insulin he is given a training program on how to inject the insulin subcutaneously in a sterile fashion. Giving yourself an injection is not a painful procedure. The needles are small and short and most people have enough injection sights to make this very easy. It is amazing how easily patients adapt to giving themselves these injections. The diabetic who has cataracts or glaucoma, though, has a special problem because he cannot read the amount of insulin indicated on the syringe. He therefore must have assistance from his relatives. I think a patient gets a tremendous amount of pride out of giving his own insulin. How much insulin you need and what type you need is determined by frequent consultation with your doctor in the early stages of your treatment. The patient, particularly if he is bright, often assumes a great deal of responsibilities that a doctor normally has in determining how much insulin he must use. He can do this only with frequent testing of his urine. It is dangerous for him to try to estimate his insulin requirement on the basis of how he feels. Giving too much insulin can be just as dangerous as having too little insulin. Too much insulin may cause a person to go into a coma; at the least he may develop a giddy feeling with hunger sensations and sweatiness over his body. At times he may become a little crazy or act as if he is on a "trip." This is why diabetics who take insulin should carry sugar with them at all times, in some form, whether it is a candy bar or crackers. This is why when we are trying to develop control of diabetes in the hospital we usually keep a bottle of orange juice at the bed side.

What will happen if I don't do anything about it?

People who develop diabetes in adulthood may go on for years without any treatment. However, they run the risks of increased infections, particularly boils on their skin and kidney infections. Most child diabetics and people who have severe diabetes in adulthood must have immediate consultation and care by a physician, or else they will die. Death from diabetes usually is preceded by a coma after the patient has lost a great deal of weight and fluid from his body.

Even diabetics who do take good care of themselves develop various complications. A diabetic is more prone to fattening of the arteries or hardening of the arteries, called atherosclerosis. Therefore diabetics will develop strokes and heart attacks more readily than other people. Also they are prone to gangrene in the extremities, particularly the feet. Because of the increased sugar in their blood diabetics are more prone to infections already mentioned, such as boils, kidney infections, blood infections, meningitis and pneumonia. Diabetics also have a lot of eye problems, but the most crippling are cataracts and glaucoma, which will be discussed in other chapters. Diabetics also get retinal detachment and a lot of hemorrhages in the back of the eye. Miscarriages and stillbirths are common among diabetic mothers and pregnancy in general is difficult with a diabetic mother. She must be under very careful supervision by a physician. Diabetics are also subject to Kimmelstiel-Wilson disease, a kidney condition in which the little cells that eliminate the fluid from the body develop hemorrhages and thickening of their walls. In this condition the kidney gradually is damaged to the point where it loses a lot of the body protein and fluid accumulates in various parts of the body. Diabetics also develop diseases of the nerves. They get a lot of numbness, tingling and paralysis in their hands and feet at times. I could go on but these are the most common complications of diabetes. It is easy to understand why it is the seventh cause of death.

Diverticulosis and Diverticulitis

What are diverticulosis and diverticulitis?

Diverticulosis is the formation of small pockets on the large intestine or colon. These are actually portions of the lining of the intestines that pop out into the fat pads around the colon and sometimes become filled with feces and may even become infected. When they become infected this condition is called *diverticulitis.* About five percent of the people over sixty years of age have these pockets but only about fifteen percent of the people with diverticulosis get inflammation in these pockets (diverticulitis) at some time during their lives.

What is the cause of diverticulitis?

Diverticulitis is usually due to infection. The precise cause is that a piece of stool gets caught in the pocket and can't get out and becomes hardened, and this becomes a good focus for infection, usually bacteria. The pockets themselves develop because of a weakening of the walls of the intestine but nobody really knows the exact cause. Probably in some cases it is hereditary.

What are the symptoms and signs of diverticulitis and diverticulosis?

Diverticulosis causes no symptoms at all, but when the pockets become inflamed then there is definite lower abdominal pain. Sometimes there is marked tenderness in the lower abdomen and cramps with each bowel movement. Occasionally there is constipation and at other times there is diarrhea. The patient may develop fever and chills. The signs and symptoms are very similar to appendicitis except that they occur on the left side of the abdomen instead of the right. In some cases there is nausea and vomiting.

What can I do about diverticulitis?

In most cases your doctor will prescribe an antibiotic, put you on a low residue diet, give you a bowel relaxant to keep you from getting spasms, and keep you at bed rest. He'll also want to give you a stool softener so that the feces will not jam up in the pockets or in the intestines where the pockets are. If conservative treatment such as this does not work then you must have surgery, just as a person with appendicitis must have surgery. When an operation is done for diverticulitis, it may be necessary to remove a large segment of the bowel.

What will happen if I don't do anything about it?

Most cases of diverticulitis will clear up without any treatment, but sometimes the little diverticuli will rupture and cause peritonitis and death. Some cases of diverticulitis will actually perforate into other portions of the intestine and form fistulous tracts. Sometimes they may form fistulous tracts to the skin and there will be a draining sinus on the skin where feculant material comes out. In other cases the diverticuli will rupture into the vagina and drain through that way. Occasionally the diverticuli become so numerous in one area of the bowel that the inflammation will create a constricting ring around the bowel and cause intestinal obstruction. Thus, if you have diverticulosis and you develop abdominal pain you should consult your physician for treatment immediately.

Drug Reactions

With the increasing number of drugs available today it is not surprising that many patients are developing reactions to these drugs. These reactions take three forms: allergic reactions, toxic reactions, and addictive or dependency reactions.

Allergic Reactions

Allergic reactions to drugs occur in two forms—acute and chronic. In the *acute* form, the patient may develop shock with a drop in blood pressure. He may develop severe shortness of breath with constriction of the bronchial tree (an asthmatic type of reaction). There may also be a skin reaction with giant hives all over the body. In the *chronic,* or delayed, form of drug reaction, the main manifestation may be a skin reaction with either macules or papules over the trunk and extremities and face, or hives; or there may be a fever and chills without any rash. Drugs that commonly produce allergic reactions are penicillin, sulfonamides, and many other antibiotics. The treatment of allergic reactions to drugs usually involves the administration of an antihistamine, such as Pyribenzamine, and possibly the use of epinephrine in the acute stage or ephedrine in the chronic stage. The most reliable drug for treatment for chronic reactions particularly is cortisone, which is also used in the treatment of acute reactions. These drugs are beneficial for the skin reactions, for the asthmatic reactions, and for the shock and hypotensive reactions. Occasionally you will have to be hospitalized for treatment so that oxygen and intravenous fluids can be administered concommitantly.

Toxic reactions

Drugs, of course, also have toxic effects on various organs of the body. Drugs that normally produce toxic reactions are digitalis, aspirin, Chloromycetin, anticonvulsants such as Dilantin, sedatives such as phenobarbital, and tranquilizers such as Thorazine. Digitalis produces a toxic reaction of nausea and occasionally vomiting and headache and fatigue. Aspirin may cause severe thinning of the blood and produce bleeding and cause ulceration of the intestinal tract. Chloromycetin notably drops the blood count, particularly the white count, and makes one more susceptible to infection—the very thing it is being prescribed for. Dilantin, the anticonvulsant, may cause acne of the face and tremendous difficulty with coordination and walking. Phenobarbital, of course, can sometimes produce an irritability of the nervous system, and when you withdraw from it you may even have convulsions. Tranquilizers such as Thorazine may cause rigid spasms of the body almost like what occurs in tetanus. This can be very alarming at times. The treatment of these reactions is most often just withdrawal of the drug. In Thorazine toxicity the administration of Benadryl or Cogentin may be necessary to stop the spastic reaction.

Addictive or dependency reaction

Addiction to various drugs is becoming more and more common. It is well known that it is one of our biggest problems in young people today. One should carefully distinguish between a drug that causes addiction and a drug that causes purely psychological dependency. Addicting drugs are the narcotics, such as morphine, heroin and codeine. These cause physiological dependency of the body on the drugs. Another addicting drug is alcohol. However, phenobarbital and the amphetamines (and possibly marijuana) cause a psychological dependency and the withdrawal effects are not severe. Even aspirin can cause psychological dependency.

The treatment of narcotic addiction must be performed in a center that is set up for this treatment. These centers are set up in many parts of the country; one of the oldest residential centers is in Lexington, Kentucky. Centers for the treatment of alcohol addiction have been set up also, notably in New York City. These are special centers where the addiction can be handled with occupational therapy, physiotherapy, and withdrawal therapy. The treatment of alcoholic addiction has been helped a great deal in recent years by the AA, as well as by the important drug, Antabuse. This drug, Antabuse will make a person very sick if he takes a small drink of liquor. Use of this drug must be carefully supervised by a physician.

Psychological addiction

Psychological dependency, as occurs with phenobarbital and amphetamines, can be difficult because the person sometimes refuses to get off the drug by himself. He may go from doctor to doctor getting prescriptions for these drugs. The only logical way to prevent this is for the county medical society to retain a listing of people who are psychologically dependent on these drugs, but very few county medical societies wish to carry the liabilities that are involved. Nevertheless these drugs rarely lead to any serious problems unless a person begins taking sixty to seventy pills a day. The worst thing about these drugs is that the more you take, the more your body becomes accustomed to these drugs, and the more you require—a sort of snowball reaction.

Doctors must be very careful when they prescribe a drug that they are controlling the drug intake and that the drug is really indicated. I might close by adding that in my practice I have never caused a case of narcotic addiction by the frequent administration of narcotics.

Ear Wax

What is ear wax?

Ear wax is the normal oily material created by small glands in the skin of the ear that protects you from invasion by bugs and bacteria. This wax may be secreted in such large quantities that it obstructs the ear and may cause hearing loss and discomfort. Many people suffer from excessive accumulation of earwax. They dig at it themselves with Q-tips that they buy at the store, or with toothpicks and other objects. They may perforate their eardrums. This should be condemned! Removal of ear wax should be done only by your doctor.

What are the symptoms and signs of ear wax?

Hearing loss, pressure and even earache are often signs of ear wax.

What can I do about it?

You should not clean your ears with anything smaller than your finger. Use of Q-tips should be discouraged completely. Use your finger to clean the outer ear. Put soap in as far as your index finger will go but no further. If you have hearing loss and earache you should see your doctor. He will see the ear wax and remove it. He can remove this if it is very thick with a special wire looped instrument. If it is soft wax, he will syringe your ear out with warm water. There is a new substance out that can dissolve the wax and he may use this to facilitate removal. You should not do it yourself.

Is ear wax dangerous?

No, ear wax is not dangerous! It is a protective device in your body against the invasion of the ear by insects or bacteria. The only thing that it could possibly do is cause hearing loss, which would be mild and rarely severe. It is only dangerous if you decide you are going to remove it.

What will happen if I don't do anything about it?

As I said, the only thing is hearing loss. You will never die of ear wax.

Emphysema

What is emphysema?

Emphysema is the trapping of air in the lungs preventing full expiration. In this condition air can get into the lungs but has difficulty getting out. This is usually due to either spasm or the collection of heavy mucus or fibrosis (growth of fibrous connective tissue) causing a constriction of the bronchial passages and partial obstruction. In irreversible emphysema the small passages of the lungs and the alveoli (little air bags that exchange the air with components in the blood) are packed up and dilated; sometimes they rupture into each other just as little balloons would rupture and become confluent. The worst thing about emphysema is that by trapping the air in the lungs it prevents the carbon dioxide from getting out of the lungs regularly and from being exhaled. The carbon dioxide accumulates in the system and may cause coma and all kinds of other disorders in the body.

What causes emphysema?

Emphysema may be caused by bronchial asthma, which is of course an allergic condition. There are many other causes. It may be caused by *silicosis* or the inhalation of other foreign elements such as coal dust or asbestos. It may be caused by repeated chronic infections to the bronchial tubes. It may also be caused by fixing of the thoracic cage due to hardening of the vertebral and rib joints. But the major cause of emphysema in our population today is *cigarette smoking.* The nicotine causes spasm of the bronchial tubes and also paralyzes the small cilia (little brushes) that sweep the bronchial tree clean of mucus, dust and bacteria. It also causes congestion of the bronchial tubes and a chronic bronchitis. There are probably other things that nicotine and tar do to the lungs that are as yet uncertain.

What are the symptoms and signs of emphysema?

The most prominent sign of emphysema is difficulty in breathing. The patient has to take twice as many breaths in order to get the same amount of oxygen and clear the same amount of carbon dioxide out of his lungs. Breathing is labored. Occasionally there is audible wheezing. In advanced cases the chest gets blown up like a barrel because of the inability to exhale all the air in the lungs. There is usually a chronic cough. This may be dry or productive of thick mucus, which is occasionally green but it is usually white or yellowish. In addition the patient may develop blue lips, nails, and skin, normally referred to as cyanosis. When the emphysema becomes severe the patient loses weight. He may lapse into coma periodically because of carbon dioxide intoxication in his body. He may become bedfast. If it is really severe the right side of his heart fails and the blood backs up into the liver, which becomes enlarged, and into the legs, causing swelling. People with emphysema are especially susceptible to pneumonia or the common cold. It is often an infection that pushes these people over from a compensated emphysema to severe respiratory difficulty and failure.

What can I do about emphysema?

You can stop smoking for one thing and also avoid any other irritating gases either in your job or elsewhere. If you live in a large city where there is tremendous pollution then you should move to the country. It is also wise to change your climate if your emphysema is related to asthma. Most of all you must stop smoking. Changing your occupation if you work around smoke or other irritants is very important. Of course you should first determine whether your occupation has anything to do with your emphysema. In states where there is a black lung program the first thing most patients do with emphysema is seek a disability claim rather than stop smoking. There is much that can be done in addition to throwing away your cigarettes to restore your lungs. Your doctor will often prescribe an expectorant (cough syrup) to loosen the thick mucus in your lungs. If he senses there might be an infection he will have a culture done and give you the appropriate antibiotics. Some patients take antibiotics regularly to prevent any infection. Your doctor may prescribe a bronchodilator or a pill like adrenalin that can keep the muscles in the bronchial tubes from going into spasm.

More important than that in severe emphysema is the intermittent positive pressure machine. This machine can force air into the lungs under pressure and thus clean out the carbon dioxide trapped in the air sacs. Usually there is a liquid mixed in the air by the machine before it is forced into the lungs, and this liquid contains an adrenalin-like substance that will dilate the bronchial passages. Sometimes the liquid contains a substance that will dissolve the mucus. Many patients find that they cough up a tremendous amount of mucus after a treatment with these machines. Fortunately now Meade Johnson Pharmaceutical Company has put a cheap intermittent positive pressure machine and nebulizer on the market that sells for under fifty dollars. Anybody can get one of these machines for home use. When the patient is in severe respiratory failure from pulmonary emphysema he may require hospitalization for continuous use of one of these machines with a good concentration of oxygen. He may even require a tracheotomy.

Is emphysema dangerous?

I think from the above discussion you can tell that it is a very dangerous condition. It is one of the ten top killers in America today.

What will happen if I don't do anything about it?

Well, you will almost certainly die of emphysema or one of its complications. Its complications include pneumonia, right heart failure, and rupture of one of the air sacs causing collapse of the lung. Emphysema is a horrible way to die. That is why I advise everybody who smokes to stop smoking to prevent this terrible disease.

How can I prevent myself from getting emphysema?

The best thing to do is to stop smoking. If you haven't started smoking then don't start. If you have bronchial asthma make sure you get adequate treatment for every attack. Get desensitized to prevent further attacks if this is possible. People who work in the mines should change their occupation. Of course, this is not always possible because of the need for the job. You can move to a dry temperature climate.

Keep your house at the same temperature or near that temperature at all times. Get flu shots every year and of course if you have early emphysema it may be wise for you to take an antibiotic the year round, just as rheumatic fever victims take penicillin to prevent another attack.

Fever Blisters

What are fever blisters?

Fever blisters are groups of little fluid-filled bubbles on the skin that usually occur on the mouth, the forehead, the nose and sometimes around the genitalia. They are very common. They are often precipitated by a cold, high fever, too much sunlight, or too much exposure to cold.

What is the cause of fever blisters?

The cause of fever blisters is a virus called herpes simplex. As I mentioned before, a cold, high fever, sunlight or exposure to too much cold weather will bring them on. They are more frequent in women around the time of menstruation.

What are the symptoms and signs of fever blisters?

The signs of a fever blister are merely tiny bubbles containing fluid on the skin. These are smaller than blisters resulting from trauma or burns. They are sometimes very painful. If they are on the face they make you feel ugly.

What can I do about a fever blister?

The best thing to do is to leave it alone. Various ointments and creams have been brought out that are supposed to heal fever blisters. Cortisone cream may give good results. Plain zinc oxide is also a very good treatment.

What can I do to prevent them?

The virus of herpes simplex cannot be wiped out completely by anything given by mouth, but if one takes smallpox injections repeatedly this may cut down on the incidence of the fever blisters. In addition, women who are in the menopause seem to be benefited by taking estrogen (hormone) supplements. Another important way of preventing them is not to be exposed to excess cold, sunlight or high fevers.

What will happen if I don't do anything about it?

If you don't do anything about a fever blister it will probably go away within a week or ten days. It is rare for it to cause any complications. There is a form of encephalitis from the herpes simplex virus, but this usually occurs in rundown people. If the herpes occurs on the eye you must get treatment by an ophthalmologist immediately. There is a new drug out called Stoxil, which is very beneficial for herpes simplex of the eye.

Fractures

There are some general remarks about all fractures that I would like to make before discussing any fractures specifically.

A fracture is any break in the continuity of a bone. This break may be completely through the bone or it may be incomplete (sometimes called a greenstick fracture). When the fracture is completely through the bone the fracture pieces may be dislocated from each other, in which case the fracture is called a "fracture dislocation." In addition there may be many fragments of bone in the fracture. Then it is called a comminuted fracture. Sometimes the fracture breaks the skin and the bone, which can be seen piercing out through the skin. This is called an open or compound fracture. Most fractures are closed fractures. The vast majority of fractures are uncomplicated closed and often incomplete fractures, which require only a cast applied in the emergency room in the hospital, and treatment can be administered on an ambulatory basis. Therefore, as you can see, most fractures are not serious.

Now I would like to discuss individual fractures and their management.

Skull fracture

The vast majority of skull fractures can be treated conservatively without operation or other procedures. It is not necessary to put a cast on, and in most cases after a few days of hospitalization for observation of the more serious complications of a head injury, the patient can be sent home. A followup x-ray is often performed three to six weeks after the fracture. In a few cases the fractured piece of bone is depressed onto the brain surface, and therefore the patient must be taken to the operating room and the piece of depressed bone lifted and possibly removed. Here again there is usually no serious complication following this type of surgery.

Fractures of the jaw

This type of fracture can be serious because, of course, we need to chew, and if the fracture is not set properly we will not be able to masticate (chew) properly. A dental surgeon usually manages this type of fracture very well. The convalescent period is long because the jaw has to be wired and chewing must be stopped and all food must be in a liquid form.

Fractures of the cervical spine (neck)

These are the most dangerous fractures because the fragment of bone may compress the spinal cord and even sever it. This will cause paralysis of the arms or legs or both. When the patient is suspected of having a broken neck his head must be handled with a great deal of care by professionals. He should not be moved until professionals arrive on the scene. Then he can be taken to the hospital where special traction is applied to the head to keep the fragments from pinching the spinal cord. Often it takes several months before healing is complete, and if there is damage to the spinal cord then these patients must have prolonged rehabilitation as well.

Fracture of the ribs

These usually require no specific treatment other than wearing a rib belt to prevent the chest from expanding and causing pain. Occasionally a broken rib may rupture the pleura of the lung, but this is rare and your doctor will know this immediately. It is unusual to have to set these fractures with the open technique.

Fractures of the wrist

With fractures of the wrist it is usually possible to set the bones under a general anesthetic in the outpatient department, and the patient may be discharged shortly after that. Sometimes a fracture dislocation is so severe that an open reduction is necessary, but this is rare.

Fracture of the shoulder

Fractures of the shoulder may often be handled by simply casting the arm to provide weight to stretch the shoulder and relocate the displaced head of the humerus. Fractures of the clavicle can be handled usually by a T-split, although occasionally they require open reduction.

Fractures of the fingers and toes

Fractures of the fingers and toes can be handled by a simple splint applied in the outpatient department. Convalescence is uneventful.

Fractured hip

This fracture occurs most often in elderly people. It is not certain whether the fracture comes first, causing trauma, or whether the fracture follows a softening of the bone and trauma. Many of these cases can now be handled by removal of the head of the hipbone or femur and replacement by a hip prosthesis (artificial bone). This means that you get a new "ball" to place in the socket. Some hips are still being nailed, and occasionally fractures of the hip must be treated by prolonged traction in the hospital for four to six months. Convalescence from these fractures is necessarily long because they occur in elderly people who heal slowly. Healing in the hip takes place slowly even in younger people.

I'm sure there are many other fractures that you wish to know about, but they are not common enough to be discussed here.

Gall Bladder Trouble

What is gall bladder trouble?

Gall bladder trouble usually means an inflammation of the gall bladder or stones in the gall bladder, which of course would eventually lead to inflammation. Rarely gall bladder trouble is due to cancer. A very frequent disorder in the United States, gall bladder trouble occurs in five to ten percent of adults.

What causes gall bladder trouble?

No one knows just how gall stones form in the gall bladder, but there is considerable investigation underway to find out. Gall stones may be made up of cholesterol, calcium bilirubinate, or calcium carbonate. There may be a single stone or several, and they may vary in size from one to two millimeters up to about two to three inches in diameter. Inflammation of the gall bladder may occur with or without stones but usually occurs with stones. If there is inflammation without the stones it may be caused by streptococcus or other bacteria. Sometimes there are no bacteria involved at all. It is only in older people that cancer of the gall bladder is found. It is not certain whether stones eventually lead to cancer.

What are the signs and symptoms of gall bladder trouble?

When there is an acute episode of gall bladder trouble the person gets severe pain in the right upper portion of the abdomen associated with nausea and vomiting. Often there is a temperature elevation. This pain often will travel through to the back or to the right shoulder blade. If the trouble is severe enough there will be jaundice. When the gall bladder trouble is of a chronic nature or if there is a milder acute attack the person may only experience mild pain in the right upper side of the abdomen along with a little nausea; he may have this only upon eating fatty foods, because fatty foods cause contraction of the gall bladder.

What can I do about gall bladder trouble?

Obviously if you have any of the symptoms mentioned above you should see your doctor immediately. Do not play around! Attacks of nausea and vomiting without pain in the abdomen are usually due to viral gastroenteritis, and if you don't have severe pain you may delay seeing your doctor, unless, of course, the nausea and vomiting continue. But if you develop jaundice or severe pain in the right upper side of your abdomen you must call a doctor immediately. He will put you in the hospital, give you intravenous fluids, put a tube down into your stomach, and give you antibiotics to reduce the inflammation of the gall bladder.

Once your temperature is down and you are feeling a little bit better he will order an x-ray of your gall bladder, called a cholecystogram (see page 282). In this case you take ten to fourteen tablets of dye and the following day pictures are taken of your gall bladder. If the gall bladder is severely diseased the dye will not be taken up by the gall bladder at all and there will be nothing seen in the x-rays. In less severe disease the dye will be concentrated in the gall bladder and the stones that are causing the trouble will be noted. Occasionally the symptoms are so severe that you must be operated on immediately before undergoing these diagnostic tests. However, usually we like to delay the operation until a definite diagnosis of gall bladder disease is made. As soon as stones are diagnosed an operation called a cholecystectomy will be performed. It is foolish to delay surgery when definite gall stones are found, particularly the smaller variety, because they will invariably lead to trouble in the future if the person lives long enough.

Is this a dangerous condition?

Silent gall stones without any symptoms are not in themselves a dangerous condition, but they may lead to severe inflammation of the gall bladder with rupture of the gall bladder and peritonitis. If a stone passes from the gall bladder down into the ducts draining the liver and the gall bladder, severe jaundice will develop and infection will spread from the gall bladder up into the liver. The person will often die from this complication. Occasionally the gall stones will eat through the wall of the gall bladder and perforate into the intestinal tract, where the larger ones will obstruct the intestines and cause severe nausea and vomiting and dehydration. This is why I feel that gall stones should be taken care of as soon as they are diagnosed.

How can I prevent myself from getting gall stones?

There is no known way of preventing gall stones with certainty, but keeping yourself on a low cholesterol, low fat diet will probably be one of the best ways. In children with hemolytic anemia it is very important to avoid too many transfusions.

Glaucoma

What is glaucoma?

Glaucoma is a condition in which the pressure in the eye is increased. The eyeball is a tight capsule that contains fluid. If the veins in the eye are unable to drain the fluid from the eye properly then the pressure in the eye increases. This may affect one or both eyes and it may be acute or chronic. It also may be congenital. It usually affects people over thirty-five years of age and is common in diabetics. A chronic form may come on very insidiously without any symptoms, but the acute form usually produces a lot of symptoms. It is estimated that at least thirty thousand people in this country are blind as a result of glaucoma.

What are the signs of glaucoma?

The signs of glaucoma in the chronic form are very few except for gradual loss of sight, usually in the peripheral area of vision. This is why it is important for people over thirty-five to have their eyes tested for acuity, for the pressure of the eye, and for the field of vision by either their medical doctor or an ophthalmologist at least every two years. There is often a hereditary history of glaucoma. The acute form of glaucoma often begins with severe pain in the eye, frontal headache, acute blurring of vision, and halos or rainbows around the visual field. There may be smarting or redness of the eye too. In congenital glaucoma the child complains of tearing and itching and sometimes headaches.

What can I do about glaucoma?

The treatment for chronic glaucoma is systemic drugs, such as diuretics and eyedrops, to keep the pupil constricted so that the fluid may escape easily through the channels near the iris. In the acute form, however, drugs and eyedrops may not be successful and a surgeon must be called in to help drain the eye with a special operation. The chronic form may also necessitate an operation in the later stages.

What will happen if I don't do anything about it?

The chances are that you will wind up blind. In the chronic form it may take several years before you are blind but in the acute form you may become blind in a few days.

How can I prevent it?

The best way to prevent glaucoma is to get a yearly or at least biennial check-up of your eyes, including a measurement of the tension in the eyeball with an instrument called a tenometer.

Goiter and Thyroid Trouble

What is goiter?

A goiter is an enlarged thyroid—the gland located on either side of the trachea just below the larynx, in a man close to the Adam's apple.

What causes it?

Some cases of goiter are associated with an overactive or underactive thyroid but frequently there is no disturbance of thyroid function at all. Many cases are due to a deficiency of iodine in the diet. The latter type is associated with the largest thyroid glands on record—sometimes the size of a grapefruit. Finally a few cases of goiter are due to cancer.

What are the symptoms and signs of goiter?

If there is an associated overactive or underactive thyroid then the symptoms mentioned under these headings (page 170) will be present. Otherwise there may be no symptoms other than the enlargement. However, if the gland gets too big it may compress the windpipe, causing choking, or compress the esophagus (food pipe) causing difficulty swallowing.

What can I do about it?

If you have no other symptoms except the enlargement you don't have to do anything, in most cases. It is wise to have your physician check it for cancer. When there are symptoms from compression of the windpipe or food pipe, the goiter should be removed surgically. Those cases associated with an overactive or underactive thyroid should be treated according to the recommendations in those sections (pages 171-72).

Is goiter dangerous?

If due to an overactive thyroid or cancer it certainly is. Also it is dangerous when it compresses the windpipe.

How can I prevent myself from getting it?

Be sure you have adequate iodine in your diet. Since salt is iodized today you will probably get enough iodine if you use salt liberally. However if you use no salt at all a vitamin with iodine added should be taken.

THE OVERACTIVE THYROID

What is an overactive thyroid?

An overactive thyroid is a thyroid that produces too much hormone. This is a fairly common endocrine disease, although it is not as common as an underactive thyroid.

What causes an overactive thyroid?

The cause is not always known but frequently an emotional upset can precipitate an overactive thyroid. There seems to be a hereditary association of thyroid disease. Occasionally there is a small benign tumor of the thyroid, but this is rarely the cause. It is almost unheard of for an overactive thyroid to be caused by a malignant tumor of the thyroid.

What are the signs and symptoms of an overactive thyroid?

Probably most people think that the most common sign of an overactive thyroid is a large thyroid gland. This, however, is not always present, although it is present in the majority of cases of an overactive thyroid. Additional symptoms that are more prominent are bulging eyes, rapid heart beat, loss of weight, and a ravenous appetite, along with frequency of urination and a desire to drink a lot of water. Fatigue mentioned in underactive thyroid is also present in an overactive thyroid. The skin becomes smooth. The nails tend to break easily and become ridged and thickened. There is a tremor of the hands, although it is a very fine tremor and often not noticed by the patient. Occasionally the patient has diarrhea. Menstrual periods seem to be scanty. The patient is often very nervous, at times depressed and at other times very elated.

What can I do about it?

There are three ways to treat an overactive thyroid. One is with drugs taken by mouth over a period of a year and one-half. These are called anti-thyroid drugs. They have certain side effects and therefore must be managed carefully by your family physician. Unfortunately, only fifty percent of patients who are treated this way are cured of their overactive thyroid. For the other fifty percent taking the medicine for a year and one-half yields no effect, except that the thyroid is controlled while the patient is on this medicine.

The second most common method used today is radioactive iodine. This is given by mouth in one calculated dose. It is successful in seventy to eighty percent of cases with the first dose and in one hundred percent of cases with subsequent doses. However, the risk of producing an underactive thyroid increases with each subsequent dose. The danger of this drug is that twenty to twenty-five percent of patients develop an underactive thyroid as a result of this treatment and must take thyroid hormone for the rest of their lives. However it is not a serious problem to have to take a thyroid tablet once a day. Therefore, I feel that this is probably the preferred method of treatment in most cases of overactive thyroid. While we haven't got enough statistics in to be sure that this radioactive material does not cause cancer it apparently doesn't.

Surgery, of course, results in a cure in at least ninety percent of cases. However, surgery gives rise to additional dangers, such as taking out the parathyroid glands, which are responsible for keeping the right amount of calcium in the body, cutting the nerve that leads to the vocal cords, and severe bleeding. A skilled surgeon, however, almost never has these complications.

Is it dangerous?

This is a very dangerous condition and if left untreated you will almost certainly die of heart failure within six months to two years.

What can I do to prevent it?

Avoiding prolonged emotional stress is about the only thing we know that possibly can prevent an overactive thyroid.

THE UNDERACTIVE THYROID

What is an underactive thyroid?

A lot of patients come to my office with the idea that they have an underactive thyroid. This is not frequently the case. There are probably as many people taking thyroid pills who have a normal thyroid as there are people on relief who could get a job. Many people who are overweight think their thyroid is underactive. Actually, only about two to three percent of obese people turn out to have an underactive thyroid. Nevertheless, an underactive thyroid is probably one of the most common endocrine diseases. An underactive thyroid does not mean one has a lump in his neck. Most frequently one does not feel anything at all in the neck of a patient who has an underactive thyroid.

What causes an underactive thyroid?

The cause of an underactive thyroid in most cases is unknown, but auto-immune disease has recently been found to be a common cause. This is a condition in which the body makes antibodies against its own thyroid tissue. Sometimes the thyroid gland simply wears out and atrophies early in one's life. Contrary to popular belief too little iodine is not the cause of an underactive thyroid. The body has a marvelous means of getting as much iodine as it can out of the smallest amount ingested.

What are the symptoms and signs of an underactive thyroid?

Since thyroid hormones are important to the metabolism of each cell in the body, somehow making them able to utilize sugar and oxygen, the result of too little thyroid hormone is simply a slowing down of the function of the tissues in all parts of the body. Thus one finds that he gets depressed and his thought processes are slower. He becomes constipated and urinates less frequently. Menstrual periods become irregular and sometimes increased bleeding occurs. He becomes fatigued, lacks energy, and sometimes experiences sore muscles. The heart slows down (beats much less frequently). There is a tendency to retain fluid in the body, although not usually in the circulatory system or the subcutaneous tissues. As I stated before, obesity is not usually associated with hypothyroidism. A hypothyroid person may put on a modest ten to twenty pounds but more than that is unusual. In infants and children, in addition to the slowing down of thoughts, mental retardation, and fatigue, there is also retarded growth of the bones. This can be observed on x-rays as a delayed ossification of the epiphysis of the bones. Children whose thyroid fails to function from birth on are called cretins.

What can I do about it?

Treatment of an underactive thyroid today is very simple. There are actually excellent preparations of thyroid hormones available, some natural and some synthetic. By simply taking one tablet a day of whatever strength your doctor feels is necessary, you can relieve all your symptoms and live a completely normal life. But before the treatment is prescribed it is very important to have a laboratory diagnosis of an underactive thyroid. The basal metabolic rate used to be the only means of diagnosing thyroid disease. Now we have several blood tests that are much more accurate. The diagnosis of thyroid disease approaches ninety-five percent accuracy. The most important tests are the T-3 Uptake, T-4 Uptake and Free Thyroxine. These tests are not easily influenced by ingestion of iodine or the special iodine dyes that are used to diagnose gall bladder and kidney disease, which do affect the protein-bound iodine, one of the older blood tests. Another useful test is a scan of the thyroid gland after the ingestion of radio-isotope material (see page 286). Your doctor will be able to decide which of these tests is most valuable for you.

One thing you must realize is that once you have been

diagnosed as having an underactive thyroid by these excellent laboratory methods you should continue to take your thyroid medicine for the rest of your life. I am amazed at some patients who take their thyroid pills, start to feel better, and decide they do not need the medicine anymore. Unless we can transplant somebody else's thyroid into your body then you must continue to take the medicine. A person with an underactive thyroid who does not get thyroid medicine can live but will feel miserable all his life.

Hay Fever

What is hay fever?

The term *hay* fever is a misnomer, because actually hay fever refers to an allergic condition of the nose and sinuses due not just to hay but most often to pollens of grass, ragweed, goldenrod, etc. In this type of condition nasal membranes and sinus membranes swell and secrete a thick white mucus. It usually occurs on a seasonal basis, although if it is due to house dust it may occur all year around.

What causes hay fever?

As mentioned above hay fever is most often caused by an allergic reaction to the pollen of goldenrod, ragweed and other grasses, trees, house dust, or by the dander of animals such as dogs and cats. There are many other substances that may cause hay fever.

What are the symptoms and signs of hay fever?

The most common symptom of hay fever is sneezing. The nose may block up forcing a person to breathe through his mouth. There is also a thick white discharge from the nose and the eyes may water. While there is no fever or chills, the person may feel general discomfort and fatigue. Occasionally there are headaches as well. Sinuses may be affected secondary to the allergy and cause a temperature on that basis.

What can I do about hay fever?

The best thing to do is to have sensitivity tests performed to determine which one of the pollens you are allergic to. Once this has been established you may receive desensitization with weekly or biweekly shots of the offending pollen, gradually increasing the amounts. This may be undertaken prior to the season in which you get the hay fever, or it may be undertaken while you have the hay fever. If this form of therapy is unsuccessful then it is necessary for your doctor to give antihistamines and nasal sprays as well as possibly cortisone to prevent the symptoms of hay fever. A very important means of combatting hay fever is an air purifier in your home. These cost about $90.00 to $100.00 and are well worth while, because they electronically remove the pollens and dust from the air. Of course, if your hay fever is due to a dog or cat it would be wise to get rid of the animal.

Is it dangerous?

Hay fever is not dangerous in itself but it may contribute to infection of the sinuses and it may eventually progress to asthma, which is more dangerous.

How can I prevent myself from getting hay fever?

The best thing to do is to stay away from the offending pollens. Do not venture into the country if you are allergic to pollens from grass or goldenrod. Stay away from the dogs or cats if you are allergic to dog or cat dander and keep your house free from dust. The purchase of an electronic air purifier is well worth while. Desensitization may be considered as a form of prevention although it is usually considered a treatment as well.

Heart Attack

What is a heart attack?

The term "heart attack" is ordinarily used by the layman to signify an acute attack of pain in the chest due to acute damage to the heart, requiring hospitalization and treatment. Most people who are told they have had a heart attack have actually suffered either partial or complete *occlusion* (blocking) of the coronary arteries by a *thrombosis* (blood clot) with subsequent damage to the heart muscle. That damage to the heart muscle may be large, or it may be small enough to be microscopic. In most cases it is as large as a quarter or half dollar.

The process that leads to occlusion of the coronary arteries is the gradual accumulation of fat deposits on these arteries, known as *atherosclerosis.* At this point we might mention the fact that atherosclerosis is related to heredity, overeating, smoking, nervous tension, and lack of exercise. As you can see, many of these causes are preventable. When the fat on the artery increases to a point where the channel through the artery is very narrowed, a clot may form because the blood slows down and can barely squeeze through the hole. Before the clot occurs the patient may experience attacks of severe pain, which last only thirty to sixty seconds. This is commonly called angina. Once the clot occurs there is usually complete loss of oxygen and sugar to a portion of the heart muscle (myocardium) and that portion dies, or becomes *infarcted.* In this case the chest pains last much longer, for two to three hours up to four days. This is the type of heart attack that requires hospitalization.

More than ten million people of all ages have some sort of heart or blood vessel disease. Heart attacks are the leading cause of death in this country.

Some people are told they have a heart attack or tell others that they have had a heart attack when actually they have merely suffered a sudden block or arrest of the heart beat, called Stokes-Adams disease (page 60). Some have had an episode of rapid heart beat, associated with sweating, occasional chest pain, and palpitations, which is called either atrial or ventricular *tachycardia.* Some people who say they have a heart attack may actually have *heart failure,* which means the heart can no longer push the blood out at the rate necessary to supply the needs of the body so that the blood backs up into the lungs and legs and causes fluid there. I am not going to discuss these types of "heart attacks" in this chapter.

What are the symptoms and signs of a heart attack?

If the heart attack is merely due to a narrowing of the lumen (central tube) of the coronary artery, then the symptoms of chest pain are not nearly so long as they are in a complete occlusion of the coronary artery by a clot with subsequent damage to the heart muscle. But the character of the pain is the same in both cases. Usually the pain is located beneath the sternum, or the center of the chest, and is a pressure-like pain as if somebody were standing on your chest. The pain may radiate into the jaw, neck or down the left or right arm. There is usually associated sweating and a weak and fatigued feeling. Sometimes there is also nausea and vomiting. The pain may go through to the back. If the blood pressure lowers significantly during the attack the patient feels dizzy and confused. If these symptoms persist more than sixty seconds then it is most likely that damage to the heart will occur and a doctor must be consulted immediately. A coronary occlusion is a dangerous condition. A person may die at any time after five minutes of this type of pain. This is why our ambulances are equipped with special equipment to treat the complications of heart attack.

What can I do about a heart attack?

As soon as you have had your first attack of chest pain described above, even if it is only for sixty seconds, you must consult your physician. He will hospitalize you and most likely place you in what we call the coronary or intensive care unit. Here there is special equipment to fight the complications of a heart attack. The most important treatment of a heart attack is bed rest. This allows the heart to beat at the lowest possible rate and stroke volume so that it does the least work. This is very important while the heart muscle is healing. Healing of the heart muscle takes from three to six weeks, just as an open wound on your skin would. Of course, if you get a deep cut of your skin you usually have sutures placed in it so that it takes only eight to ten days to heal. However we cannot open the heart of a patient with a heart attack and remove the dead material and suture the heart together. If during your period of healing the heart wall should weaken enough to force a rupture, then a surgeon may be called in to sew up this rupture but this is usually not the case.

During the first three days of healing the heart is very vulnerable to what we call *arrhythmias*. These arrhythmias are really the development of a series of extra beats in your heart, occasionally making the rate go to three or four hundred per minute. Because it goes so fast in some cases the branches of the heart muscle do not contract together causing what we call a cardiac arrest with ventricular fibrillation (quivering). In this case the heart might as well not be beating at all, because the effective movement of blood through the heart stops. The nurse will then apply a machine called the defibrillator, which causes a shock to go through the heart to completely relax the heart muscle for a short period so that it will all start beating together simultaneously. At least a fifth of the patients that are admitted to the coronary care unit may go into an arrhythmia of some kind and one out of ten might require the use of the defibrillator. To prevent the patient from going into these arrhythmias, the minute that the nurse spots extra beats on the oscilloscopic monitor (which is placed on each patient in a coronary care unit) she starts drugs intravenously to suppress them.

In addition to these measures aimed at preventing complications of a heart attack, during your hospital stay in the coronary care unit you will also be given oxygen continuously to limit the amount of damage to your heart and make your heart do less work. You will often be given a blood thinner to prevent further clotting of your coronary arteries and possibly to dissolve the clot. The blood thinner may be continued for months or even years after you are discharged from the hospital, depending on your age and other factors. (You must also stop smoking and refrain from eating too much.)

Of course, to you the most important part of the treatment is eliminating the pain. Morphine is usually given for this. Most patients stay in the coronary care unit at least three to six days. After that they remain in the hospital for at least two weeks more and perhaps up to six weeks more.

Another complication that is less discussed is cardiac arrest, an actual stopping of the heart beat. In other words the heart will slow down to thirty to forty beats a minute and then stop altogether. In this case a *pacemaker* must be applied to induce an electrical discharge over the heart every second so that the heart will contract sixty or more times per minute. This pacemaker may be attached to the arm with a wire from it inserted into the vein and threaded directly into the heart. Or the pacemaker may be placed inside the skin on a more permanent basis with the wires connected directly to the muscle of the heart. In either case this is a vital little machine to keep your heart beating. We are very proud of the advances that have been made in the past ten years in the treatment of heart attacks. The death rate has dropped precipitously because of excellent treatment in coronary care units and even out in the hospital wards.

It is very important after the patient gets out of the hospital that he be allowed to rest, not go upstairs too frequently for at least six to eight weeks after leaving the hospital, and have regular periods of light exercise every day. The diet must be low in cholesterol and fat, and overeating at any meal is to be discouraged. The patient must not smoke for the rest of his life and must avoid nervous tension at all cost. Remember, the coronary occlusion that produced the heart attack has not been removed during the hospital stay. Therefore another piece of heart muscle supplied by the artery could become damaged if too much stress is placed on the heart.

What will happen if I don't do anything about my heart attack?

Two-thirds of people who do not do anything about a heart attack may live but the other third will certainly die of their heart attack from one of the complications mentioned above. I wouldn't want these odds!

How can I prevent myself from getting a heart attack?

The most important thing to prevent yourself from getting a heart attack would be to choose parents who have very little hardening of the arteries. In other words heredity is the most important factor that we know of in inducing atherosclerosis. If your parents did not die of a heart attack until a very late age, say seventy or eighty, or ninety, then it is unlikely that you will.

But although you can't do much about choosing your parents, you can do something about other factors. The most important factor is to stop smoking. We know that smoking increases the blood cholesterol, that it injures the arteries and veins of the body, and that it also increases the coagulability of the blood (see page 232). Your diet is very important. It is not so much what you eat (such as a low-cholesterol diet) as it is the amount you eat. Sure, a lot of us thin people think we can eat as much as we want because we do not get fat. Overloading our systems with food, however, will surely cause an increase in the blood cholesterol and this may deposit on the arteries of our bodies. Sugar and protein both can be converted into cholesterol, not just fat alone. And once cholesterol gets into the body it has very little way of getting out.

Another very important thing is to get regular exercise, not just a walk to the bus or a walk on the golf course once or twice a week. Regular planned daily exercise in the form of the Canadian Air Force exercises, or riding an exercycle for the equivalent of two to five miles a day is excellent. Playing tennis two or three times a week is an excellent form of exercise if you live in a climate that allows it or if you know where there are indoor tennis courts.

Finally, it is very important to avoid nervous tension. Don't carry a lot of problems around with you. If you can't solve a problem immediately then stop worrying about it. Go on to something else that you can do something about. If there is too much stress on your job, quit it! If your wife nags you too much then perhaps you should consult your family doctor or a psychiatrist about these problems.

For those people who have *angina pectoris,* which means that the arteries of their heart are noticeably beginning to narrow, it is wise to begin anticoagulants, as well as to observe the precautions mentioned above. There are drugs that will dilate the coronary arteries, such as nitroglycerin and its derivatives, that should be on hand at all times. In some cases they should be taken regularly. When the attacks of angina continue to occur despite the use of drugs and anticoagulants and despite following the above health habits, then an operation to remove the clot or to bypass the narrowed lumen is in order. This operation is receiving wider use today and it is proving very successful. The procedure is that a small piece of the saphenous vein in your leg is taken out and placed adjacent to the coronary artery that is narrowed so that the blood can run from the upper part of the coronary artery, around the occlusion, and through the vein graft to the lower portion of the coronary artery without any obstruction. More and more people will have this operation, even some people sixty-five years of age and over. Before this operation can be performed, however, x-rays must be taken of your heart while injecting dye into the coronary arteries so that we can find where the narrowing of the arteries is. If the narrowing is too low in the coronary artery, then the operation will not be of much value.

Hemorrhoids

What are hemorrhoids?

Hemorrhoids are varicose veins of the rectum. These are dilated veins that project outside the anal canal and sometimes may be as large as grapes. They are not usually large except during a bowel movement.

What is the cause of hemorrhoids?

Frequently hemorrhoids are hereditary. However, hemorrhoids may be caused by pregnancy, particularly with a prolonged gestational period or when the head of the fetus is pressing posteriorly against the rectum. In addition hemorrhoids may be caused by constipation.

What are the symptoms and signs of hemorrhoids?

The most common symptom of hemorrhoids is frequent bleeding with the stools. This is usually bright red bleeding. There may also be pain at the time of moving the bowels. The patient sometimes feels a lump, particularly at the time of moving the bowels. If the hemorrhoid contains a thrombosis then the lump will be present even between bowel movements and there will be a great deal of pain constantly. There is a tremendous fear of moving the bowels because this accentuates the pain so much.

What can I do about hemorrhoids?

The best thing to do about hemorrhoids is to take a stool softener such as mineral oil or roughage such as carrots and other vegetables to keep the stools soft. You must not get constipated because this will only aggravate the hemorrhoids. A regular bowel movement every day is a must for a person who has hemorrhoids. However, I do not recommend taking laxatives as a means of maintaining regularity. The doctor can prescribe a stool softener that may be slightly better than mineral oil. Once the hemorrhoids start bleeding or become extremely painful then you should see your doctor. If he discovers a clot in the hemorrhoid he will incise the hemorrhoid and remove the clot. If the hemorrhoids continue to bleed then surgery will have to be performed to remove them. Large hemorrhoids that bleed or clot frequently should be removed by surgery in the hospital.

Are hemorrhoids dangerous?

No. A clotted hemorrhoid will not usually move to the lung (pulmonary embolism) or cause any other serious consequences. It would be very unusual for you to bleed to death from a hemorrhoid.

How can I prevent hemorrhoids?

The best way to prevent hemorrhoids is to avoid constipation. When you are constipated do not strain at the stool so that the veins will not become distended. It is better to lubricate the rectum and take either an oil or tap water enema. If necessary break up the stool with your finger.

Hernias and Ruptures

The terms hernia and rupture actually are interchangeable. When a person speaks of having a rupture, however, he usually means that he has a rupture of the inguinal (groin) area, either with an *indirect hernia* through the inguinal ring (the little ring that provides the opening for the tube leading to the testicles) or with a *direct inguinal hernia,* i. e., a breaking down of the abdominal wall in the groin area.

However, by the term rupture the patient may mean a rupture of the belly button or a rupture of an incision in the abdominal wall causing loops of intestine to extrude through just beneath the skin. Or he may mean a rupture of a disc in his spine. Rarely he may mean a rupture of the diaphragm, but this condition is much more often referred to as a hiatal hernia. The important thing to remember from all this is that a rupture and a hernia usually mean the same thing and that they may occur in many areas. These hernias are grouped together because the treatment is usually very very similar, that is, surgery. The conditions causing them are often the same.

HIATAL HERNIA

What is a hiatal hernia?

A hiatal hernia is the dilation of the normal opening in the diaphragm that allows the esophagus (the tube leading from the mouth to the stomach) to pass through into the stomach. This hole is ordinarily a half-inch to one inch in diameter but when it becomes herniated it may reach between two and five inches in diameter. If this occurs then the stomach may slide up into the chest, either alongside the esophagus or with the esophagus.

What causes a hiatal hernia?

A hiatal hernia is often congenital; thus, if you have it there is a good possibility your mother, grandmother or grandfather, etc., had it, too. Or it may be produced by a severe blow to the abdominal wall, by an occupation that requires straining a good deal, and by other traumatic conditions.

What are the symptoms and signs of hiatal hernia?

The most common symptom of a hiatal hernia is heartburn. This usually occurs after meals and sometimes may occur one half hour before meals; it is frequently brought on by lying down. The heartburn may be increased by deep breathing or by coughing. There is often regurgitation of food up to the mouth and there may also be a lot of gas. Vomiting may occur but that is rare. Sometimes the first sign of a hiatal hernia is blood in the stool, either black or fresh blood. This is due to ulceration of the lining of the esophagus.

What can I do about it?

Once your doctor has made a diagnosis of a hiatal hernia by administering a barium swallow, or an upper GI series or by esophagoscopy, he will then prescribe a diet consisting mainly of milk, soft foods, and antacids, such as Maalox or Gelusil. The most important thing he will ask you to do is elevate the head of your bed on six-inch blocks. This will keep the acid in your stomach (and also your stomach) from moving up into your chest when you are lying down and sleeping at night. If these measures fail then you must have surgery. The surgery for hiatal hernia is no more difficult than that for removal of gall bladder, so you have nothing to fear.

Is it dangerous?

Hiatal hernia is not dangerous. Many people live a pretty normal life with it. It may cause ulceration of the esophagus with bleeding, in which case you can bleed to death, but this is unusual. Occasionally the ulceration may become severe enough to cause a stricture of the esophagus, making it difficult to swallow your food. It is very unusual for the esophagus to ulcerate all the way through (perforate). I have treated at least eighty percent of my patients with hiatal hernia conservatively with a bland diet and elevation of the head of the bed.

How can I prevent a hiatal hernia?

The best way to prevent a hiatal hernia is to take a job where there is very little lifting or strain. Most of us cannot do this because we are trained for a certain type of work and must continue with it. If one already has a hiatal hernia, in order to prevent the complications it may be wise to switch to a white collar job, even if it requires retraining. Keeping the head of the bed elevated will prevent serious complications.

INGUINAL HERNIA

What is an inguinal hernia?

Inguinal hernia is (1) an enlargement of the normal hole through which pass the tubes to the testicles from their origin near the bladder, or (2) a weakening and rupture of the abdominal wall in the vicinity of this hole. Women can have an inguinal hernia, also, but they have only small remnants of tubes passing through the inguinal ring.

What causes an inguinal hernia?

The most common cause of an inguinal hernia is congenital. Therefore, if your father, mother, grandmother or grandfather had an inguinal hernia you may have one, too. Most hereditary inguinal hernias are of the first type, or bilateral. The direct type of inguinal hernia, however, where there is weakening of the abdominal wall, may occur in obese people or in people who have to strain a good deal on their jobs lifting things. Obesity weakens the abdominal wall and makes people more susceptible to the direct type of inguinal hernia.

What are the symptoms and signs of an inguinal hernia?

You may not notice that you have an inguinal hernia unless the intestines fall down into the scrotum through the enlarged ring or the ruptured area of the abdominal wall; in that event you will feel a tremendous enlargement of your testicles. Or you may simply feel a bulge in the abdominal wall above your pubic hair. There is often no pain associated with the passage of the intestines down into the scrotum, but if the intestines get jammed there and you cannot push them back then you will develop pain. If the doctor cannot push them back either then we consider that your hernia has become incarcerated and surgery is mandatory. If the intestines become twisted or swollen in the scrotal sac there may be strangulation of the affected portion of the intestines, and of course this will cause severe pain. Strangulation will also cause dilatation of the abdomen, with distention, gas, and vomiting—all the symptoms of intestinal obstruction.

What can I do about an inguinal hernia?

The best thing to do is to have it operated on as soon as it is discovered. This will prevent you from having any complications, such as strangulation and intestinal obstruction. There are some people who insist on wearing a truss, which is a pad that is placed over the enlarged ring to prevent the intestinal contents from coming down into the scrotum, but this is a very poor method of treatment.

Is it dangerous?

From the many number of people that walk around with these hernias without getting them treated, it is obvious that complications are unusual. However, because the complications are serious (strangulation and intestinal obstruction), one should operate on this condition as soon as it is discovered. It is a very simple operation as long as there are no complications prior to surgery.

How do I prevent myself from getting an inguinal hernia?

The best way to prevent yourself from getting this condition is to become a white-collar worker. However, not all of us can do this and some of us must lift a hundred to two hundred pounds in our jobs. You should keep slim. If you could choose the right parents you might have a better chance of not getting this condition, too.

UMBILICAL HERNIA

Umbilical hernia is an enlargement of the ring through which the umbilical tube passes from the baby to the mother. It is through this tube that the baby gets all its nourishment from the mother while it is in the womb. Ordinarily after birth the small ring through which these tubes pass closes over, and all you have is an indentation of the skin, called the navel or umbilicus. However, if the abdominal muscles and the fibrous tissue around the opening do not close, then you are left with an umbilical hernia.

What causes an umbilical hernia?

Umbilical hernias, like other hernias, are often congenital.

What are the symptoms and signs of an umbilical hernia?

The most common symptom is usually just a bulge at the navel. This may be quite a large bulge if the intestinal contents have passed into the navel. In adults these bulges may become quite large, containing large amounts of intestines or the fatty coverings of the intestines called the omentum. If the intestines become jammed in the hernial sac then there may be severe pain, nausea, vomiting, and occasionally intestinal obstruction.

What can I do about it?

The best thing to do is to have it operated on. In some cases in infants the hole is small enough that it will close over after a year or two; but if the hernia is still present after two years of age then I feel it should be operated on. The operation is simple and does not require a very long hospital stay.

Is it dangerous?

No, this condition is not as dangerous as an inguinal hernia because strangulation of the bowel and intestinal obstruction are much less frequent. However, it can be an unsightly condition and therefore should be operated on.

How can I prevent myself from getting an umbilical hernia?

As an adult, once again, you would be less likely to get this condition if you were a white-collar worker and did not have to lift very much on your job. Also, keeping slim will help prevent this type of hernia.

FEMORAL HERNIA

What is a femoral hernia?

Femoral hernia is an enlargement of the ring through which the artery, vein and nerve to the legs pass. If this ring becomes sufficiently enlarged, then the intestines can pass down through the ring to the upper part of the leg, just as they pass into the scrotum through the enlarged inguinal ring. Fortunately, this advanced stage is pretty rare except in the elderly male.

What causes it?

Obesity in pregnancy, because it distends the abdomen and stretches the normal ring, may be the most common cause of this condition. That is why this condition is four times more frequent in women. Heredity probably plays a small role in this condition also.

What are the symptoms and signs of femoral hernia?

The most common symptom is a bulge in the groin; if the intestines have fallen down into the groin and are prevented from coming back then there may be pain. Again, if there is strangulation and swelling of the intestines there will be more pain and intestinal obstruction, just as there is in inguinal hernias and umbilical hernias.

What can I do about it?

The thing to do is to have it operated on immediately. To wear a truss in this type of hernia is ridiculous because it is more likely that there will be strangulation of the intestines if they pass through a femoral hernia.

Is it dangerous?

Yes, this is the more dangerous type of hernia and should be operated on immediately.

What can I do to prevent it?

Staying slim and avoiding pregnancy would probably be the best two things you could do to prevent this.

INCISIONAL HERNIA

Incisional hernias occur following surgery in the area of the scar. They are obviously not hereditary because they are produced by a surgeon's knife. However, they are common in obese people, whose tissues heal and scar poorly. The larger the incision made for your abdominal operation, the more chance there is for a hernia. Here again the most common symptom is a mass, which is due to the intestinal contents' getting into the incisional defect. The hernia is produced because, while the skin remains intact, the muscles fail to come back together with a neat scar. The best cure for this is immediate operation.

However, with many patients we insist that they lose weight before we perform the operation again, because we will probably have the same results if they are still overweight. This is not as dangerous a hernia as the other types mentioned above, but it should be operated on nevertheless because of its unsightly appearance and the chance of complications, such as strangulation and intestinal obstruction. The best way to prevent this type of hernia from developing is to lose weight before elective surgery and stay thin.

Hypochondriac

What is a hypochondriac?

Generally a hypochondriac is a person who complains of numerous pains and aches and other medical symptoms for which there is no physical basis. Every one of us gets aches and pains in various parts of our body from time to time, but we usually wait a couple of hours or a day or so and watch them pass by. A hypochondriac, however, is quick to bring each ache and pain to the attention of his family and his doctor. Of course, hypochondriacs get real diseases also, and therefore the doctor must examine these patients with care.

Probably a great many people consider themselves hypochondriacs who are not. This is because all of us have the aches and pains that the hypochondriac has, but we keep our fears to ourselves and do not trouble doctors as much as the hypochondriac does. Some aches and pains are justifiably frightening, and it is the physician's duty to calm you regarding these complaints. There is a great tendency in the medical profession today to label patients as hypochondriacs. It is true that over fifty percent of the patients who come to a doctor's office have relatively minor complaints, but this does not mean that their pain is not real! It does not mean that it is unimportant for the patient to find out what the cause is.

At the opposite extreme from the hypochondriac is the person who waits for months before he makes an appointment with his doctor to find out about his pain or ache. These people jeopardize their health severely because they are reluctant to see a doctor early in the course of their disease.

The hypochondriac usually has an underlying emotional problem, and this could be extremely severe. It could arise out of something that has happened in his job or marriage recently, or it could be something that dates back to his childhood. People who are severely depressed or who have schizophrenia or other psychotic disorders often have hypochondriacal complaints. Therefore the physician must be on the alert to ascertain that the hypochondriacal symptoms are not the warning of a more severe psychiatric illness requiring institutionalization. Hypochondriacs are a bonanza to the average doctor because they pay their bills and make frequent visits. Like diabetes, their emotional condition is very resistant to cure. However, many of them, if they underwent proper psychoanalysis, could be cured. Tranquilizers usually do not cure the true hypochondriac because he needs his doctor's sympathy and understanding for other reasons. Therefore he will keep coming back, regardless of what tranquilizers he is put on.

The majority of normal people may, from time to time, experience pains or aches that are entirely due to nerves, particularly when they are under a great deal of stress with their job, their marriage, their children, or their in-laws; but these people differ greatly from hypochondriacs because once they have been reassured by their physician that the cause is emotional they can usually live with the complaint or will eventually get over it with the use of tranquilizers.

Infectious Mononucleosis

What is infectious mononucleosis?

Infectious mononucleosis is an infectious disease of the blood-forming organs of the body. It affects primarily young people between the ages of thirteen and thirty. It is probably a contagious disease caused by a virus.

What is the cause of infectious mononucleosis?

As stated above, the cause of infectious mononucleosis is probably a virus. It seems that it can be spread by kissing, by sharing eating utensils, or by blood transfusions.

What are the symptoms and signs of infectious mononucleosis?

Infectious mononucleosis is usually ushered in by a fever with swelling of the lymph glands, particularly the ones next to the throat in the neck, and a sore throat. There may be a rash as well as swelling of the spleen or liver. Some patients have a mild meningitis or peripheral neuritis along with the symptoms mentioned above. Sometimes there may be abdominal pain similar to appendicitis.

What can I do about infectious mononucleosis?

Most probably you will not be certain about the diagnosis until you consult your physician. Unfortunately, while he has very adequate facilities for making the diagnosis of infectious mononucleosis, there is little that he can do in the way of treatment. Bed rest for four to six weeks and sometimes longer, as well as aspirin for severe temperatures, is the best treatment. He will perform blood tests on you to diagnose this disease. The blood count will show predominance of lymphocytes (the type of white cells that come from lymph tissue). In addition he will do an antibody tests on your blood to diagnose infectious mononucleosis. However, even if these blood tests are negative you may still have infectious mononucleosis.

Is it dangerous?

No. Infectious mononucleosis is not a dangerous disease. Very few people die of infectious mononucleosis and there are usually no serious complications.

What can I do to prevent infectious mononucleosis?

As stated above you can refrain from kissing but this is a difficult thing to do. In addition you can avoid blood transfusions unless they are definitely indicated. Other than that it would be very difficult to prevent this contagious disease.

Influenza

What is influenza?

Influenza is often referred to by people as the "flu," but when they say the "flu" they sometimes mean the intestinal flu. Influenza is the respiratory "flu" which manifests itself by runny nose, sore throat, and a cold and cough. The intestinal flu is really viral gastroenteritis and manifests itself by vomiting and diarrhea. In this chapter we are discussing the respiratory type of "flu."

What causes it?

Influenza is caused by a number of influenza viruses. These attack the respiratory tract such as the throat, nose, trachea and bronchi. Many people who come to the doctor complaining of a cold actually have influenza. Flu is a very frequent cause of the common cold. It is a common condition that occurs almost every year. This is why there is so much publicity about getting vaccinations for influenza. There are epidemics every five to ten years that wipe out large numbers of our population, but the victims are usually older people or the extremely young.

What are the symptoms and signs of influenza?

Influenza usually presents with generalized aches and pains, pain behind the eyeballs, headache, sore throat, cough, runny nose, and a temperature. Often influenza causes a dry cough. When a person finds that his cough is getting wet, particularly when the material that one coughs up is yellowish or greenish, bacterial pneumonia probably has set in on top of the influenza. This requires treatment with an antibiotic such as penicillin. There is no antibiotic that will cure influenza.

What can I do about influenza?

As I stated above there is no antibiotic that can cure influenza and the most important aspect of treatment is preventing the complications. The complications of influenza are pneumonia, sinusitis, and a bad ear infection. In order to prevent this sort of thing one should go to bed, get adequate rest, drink a lot of fluid, take aspirin, and in some cases take a nasal decongestant along with it such as Dristan. In general, antibiotics are discouraged. I would request that patients do not insist on an antibiotic or a shot of penicillin from their physician for this.

What can I do to prevent it?

Get your doctor to give you an influenza vaccine! One of the most important parts of managing this illness is preventing it in people who are most likely to get the complications, such as pneumonia. The people most likely to get this are those over sixty-five and people with cardiovascular disease, such as congestive heart failure or pulmonary emphysema. These people should all get the vaccine annually. Also extremely small infants are susceptible.

In summary

Influenza affects the respiratory tract and of itself is a short-termed illness. While it causes a lot of days missed from work it rarely kills people in good general health and rarely causes any disability. The treatment for it is symptomatic. Antibiotics are not used unless there are complications such as pneumonia, ear infection or sinusitis. People who are under sixty-five and in very good health do not require the vaccination, but this can be had from a local physician if the patient desires.

Kidney Infections and Cystitis

What causes kidney infections and cystitis?

Kidney infections and cystitis are very common in women and young girls, particularly women of the child-bearing age. The infection is common during pregnancy. At least twenty-five percent of my patients have or will have cystitis or kidney infection at one point in their lives. Kidney infection usually is called by the medical term, pyelonephritis. Most kidney or bladder infections (cystitis) are due to bacteria. It is unusual for viruses to cause clinical infection of this organ system. This type of kidney involvement does not cause dropsy (accumulation of fluid), whereas Bright's disease, or glomerulonephritis, does.

Men do not get kidney infections as frequently as women. The reason for this is obvious: the woman's bladder is very close to the outside; the little tube called the urethra that leads from the woman's bladder to the outside is very short, measuring one and one-quarter inches long, whereas the male urethra with the addition of the penis is at least three to five inches long when the penis is not erect; in addition the woman's vagina is very close to the opening of the urethra so that many bacteria that normally grow in the vagina find their way to the bladder. On top of this women are subject to the trauma of intercourse, which sometimes causes a battering of the bladder, making it more susceptible to infection. Sometimes women get infections because they wipe their bottoms the wrong way, bringing small particles of stool from the rectum up across the vagina and the opening from the bladder. The stool has a certain number of bacteria in it. One of them, E. Coli, is one of the most common causes of kidney and bladder infections.

Kidney and bladder infections may also derive from bacteria reaching them through the blood, but this is probably much less common. This route of infection is equally as common in men as in women. When a man gets a kidney infection it is often a sign that he has some other disease of the kidneys or bladder, such as a stone, cancer, or a congenital malformation. If women get repeated kidney and bladder infections they should also be considered to have one of these diseases. In this case they should have special x-ray studies, such as an intravenous pyelogram. In addition they should probably have *cystoscopy,* which involves putting a metal tube with a light on it into the bladder and having a look around for such conditions as a stone, tumor or stricture, etc. Older men have a greater incidence of kidney infections because their prostate glands enlarge and obstruct the flow of urine from the bladder through the urethra to the outside. One important cause of kidney infection in both male and female is venereal diseases such as gonorrhea. These lead to strictures of the urethra and primary infection of the prostate and urethra.

What are the symptoms and signs of a kidney or bladder infection?

With a kidney infection there may be no symptoms at all, and this is why everyone should have a frequent check of their urine especially women of child-bearing years. One urine sample may not even show pus cells or bacteria, so that sometimes it is important to inspect two or three samples. When the kidney infection does produce symptoms there is usually a chill with fever and back pain, particularly in the mid-back on one or both sides. There usually is frequency of urination, and if the kidney infection spreads to the bladder there is burning on urination. Frequently the patient will notice that the urine is cloudy, smoky or bloody. By frequency we mean that the patient goes to the bathroom at least once or twice every two hours and gets up three or four times at night to urinate. Of course old men with prostate trouble will be up frequently at night because their bladder is distended constantly and they can get only a little urine out at a time; this does not necessarily mean that they have associated kidney infection. If there is only a bladder infection there frequently is no chill and no fever, but the burning on urination is more consistent and there is often blood in the urine. Bladder infections occur commonly in newly married women because of the fact that the penis is battering the bladder and this is a new experience (we hope). It has not been proven that unusual sexual practices (such as cunnilingus) contribute to bladder infections. Pure blood in the urine does not always mean that there is cancer in the bladder or kidney, as is commonly believed. If blood appears without accompanied pain, however, this may be a first sign of cancer in older people.

What can I do about a kidney infection or cystitis?

We are fortunate that in the past thirty-five years sulfa and antibiotics have been discovered that can control almost all kidney infections. Antibiotics such as pencillin, tetracycline and the nitrofurans can be employed. Your doctor will take a special sample of your urine under very sterile conditions, put the sample in a culture tube, then lay it out on a plate to determine which drug will be most effective in the individual infection. Unlike treatment for pneumonia and respiratory infections, one must take the antibiotic or sulfa for a much longer period of time. Two weeks is the average but in resistant cases it may be necessary to continue treatment for three to six months. Some patients require a urinary antiseptic, such as Mandelamine, taken by mouth for the rest of their lives. As I said above when these symptoms recur after adequate treatment then it suggests that there are other diseases of the kidney or bladder that must be investigated. An enlarged prostate, a stone, a tumor, or a congenital malformation are just a few to look for. In these cases it is necessary that a cystoscopy and an intravenous pyelogram, described above, be performed.

What will happen if I don't do anything about it?

Frequently your symptoms will go away because the infection becomes chronic. However, when this happens the bacteria spread up into the cortex of the kidney and make little abscesses all over, and eventually the kidney becomes unable to function. If this happens to both of the kidneys you may cease to make urine and will die of uremic poison. If it happens to one kidney, that one can be removed surgically. Chronic infections of the bladder may require installations of antiseptics, such as silver nitrate, and you may have to have your ureters transplanted into the intestinal tract or onto the surface of your skin, bypassing the bladder until it heals.

How can I prevent myself from getting a kidney infection?

One very important thing is to wipe yourself in the direction from front to back instead of from back to front. Do not douche frequently. Avoid venereal disease. Be careful with your sexual technique not to cause any pain. Get yearly vaginal examinations and "pap" smears to make sure there is no cancer there. Promptly treat any infection of the kidneys or bladder so that no scars are left in the area.

Kidney Stones

What are kidney stones?

Kidney stones are not as common as people might think but they are common enough to be mentioned in a book of this type. They are more common in men than in women. These stones are usually made up of calcium oxalate, but they may be made of phosphates or uric acid, the acid that is found frequently in gout. They are more common in hot climates. This indicates that dehydration may be an important factor.

What is the cause of kidney stones?

The cause of kidney stones is for the most part unknown, but it is definite that urinary stasis (inactivity) from obstruction somewhere in the urinary tract, as from the bladder through the urethra or from the kidneys through the ureters, is a very important factor in the production of stones. Kidney infection also contributes to the production of stones. We also know that people with hyperparathyroidism (overactivity of the little glands that regulate calcium in the body) will have kidney stones. Finally, gout leads to kidney stones in a small percentage of cases.

What are the symptoms of a kidney stone?

A kidney stone will produce the most excruciating pain in either side of the body or in the back, and most people who have had it say that this is the worst pain that they have ever experienced in their lives. The pain builds up in waves to a climax and then drops off, only to repeat itself. When the stone is passed down into the bladder then there is much less pain, but there will still be some pain on voiding until the stone passes from the bladder. Usually there are no chills or fever, but these may occur if there is associated infection. In addition, one often finds that his urine is full of blood. The pain described and blood in the urine are the two main symptoms of a kidney stone.

What can I do about it?

A kidney stone will usually pass by itself as long as you drink a lot of water and go to the bathroom frequently. Seventy to eighty percent of them will pass this way. If it does not pass in a couple of days with this treatment plus some treatment to relax the muscles in the walls of the ureter, then it is necessary for the urologist to take the stone out. You will be taken to the operating room and anesthetized so that this will not be a painful procedure. He can do this either by putting an instrument up through your bladder up the ureter, crushing the stone and dragging it out, or by actually making an incision and going after the stone directly.

What will happen if I don't do anything about it?

Some people carry stones with them for years and years without having any trouble. One important thing that will happen is frequent infection. If you can stand the pain, it is unlikely that any serious damage will occur. A stricture of the ureter may occur and block your kidney, destroying it. However, your other kidney can function without it and keep you alive.

How can I prevent myself from getting stones?

X-rays of the kidney as well as cystoscopy (see page 283) should be done to determine whether other conditions in your kidney or urinary tract could be causing stones. You can exclude calcium from your diet. It would also be helpful to increase the amount of acid and fluid in your diet. Of course, if you have hyperparathyroidism or gout, then treatment of these conditions is in order.

Meningitis

What is meningitis?

Meningitis is an infection of the coverings of the brain called the meninges. These are three layers of tissue, the dura mater, the pia mater and arachnoid. They lie between the skull and brain and vertebrae and spinal cord.

What causes it?

Meningitis is caused by many bacteria, viruses, fungi and spirochetes. The most common bacteria causing meningitis are the meningococcus, influenza and pneumococcus. Tuberculosis and syphilis may also cause meningitis, but these are uncommon today. Probably the commonest form of meningitis seen today is due to a virus. Even measles and mumps virus may produce a meningitis. Viral meningitis is usually mild and nothing to worry about.

What are the symptoms and signs of meningitis?

Meningitis usually begins with a fever, generalized headache and a stiff neck. Mothers should always suspect meningitis when their children have fever and headache. However, if they can flex the head onto the chest—that is, bring the chin down to within an inch of the chest without much pain —then meningitis is very unlikely. In bacterial meningitis, confusion and coma may develop rapidly. This is also true of some forms of viral meningitis. Vomiting and focal paralysis of the muscles in the body may occur. Meningococcal meningitis may be associated with a rash.

What can I do about it?

If the only symptoms your child complains of are headache and a fever, check for a stiff neck. If it is present or there is any doubt, see your doctor at once. Naturally if your child becomes stuporous or comatose you should see your doctor immediately. He will probably do a spinal tap and if it shows pus cells or high pressure, he will hospitalize your child and start massive doses of antibiotics. These will probably be continued until cultures prove it isn't caused by a bacteria.

Is it dangerous?

Bacterial meningitis and some types of viral meningitis are life-threatening if untreated. Fortunately, antibiotics can save most cases, but you must be treated early. Most cases of viral meningitis will clear up by themselves.

What can I do to prevent it?

Stay away from crowded living quarters and crowded theaters or department stores. Some types of meningitis are spread by animals and flies, so these should be avoided. Also if you have a bad infection of the ear or sinus, or infection anywhere in the body, be sure and get treatment before it spreads to the blood and brain.

Mental Retardation

What is mental retardation?

Mental retardation is retardation in the development of intellect during childhood. Most states consider any child who fails to attain an I.Q. of 90 as mentally retarded. If it is below 80 the child is often eligible for institutionalization.

What causes it?

Most causes of mental retardation are hereditary. Many causes are due to either anoxia (lack of oxygen) or trauma during labor or birth. Babies in a breech, forceps, premature or other unusual type of delivery may suffer mental retardation. Another common cause is damage to the baby while it is being carried by the mother. This may be due to trauma, infection (such as German measles) or other as yet unknown causes. Finally congenital defects such as mongolism and jaundice of the newborn are not uncommon causes.

What are the symptoms of it?

Anyone can diagnose the severely retarded. The borderline cases are difficult and may only be picked up by the school teacher. If your child is "flunking" more than one or two subjects he should definitely be seen by a neurologist. A peculiar type of retarded child that can be recognized early is the hyperactive child. These children are into everything and actually appear very smart. They are hard to discipline because they have poor concentration powers. Most people recognize a mongoloid but a few will only be spotted by your pediatrician.

What can I do about it?

If you suspect your child has mental retardation take him to a pediatrician or neurologist. He will define the cause of the retardation and have a psychologist test the child to determine how severe it is. Many times there is no retardation at all but merely an emotional problem that can be treated by psychotherapy and tranquilizers. Occasionally a change in the child's diet (as in cases of phenylketonuria and galactosemia) may prevent further deterioration and improve the child. Occasionally an underactive thyroid is found to be the cause and treated. Drugs such as amphetamine sulfate, Ritalin and Deaner may improve the child. More important, placing the child in special education classes and brain damage classes will help him learn faster. Occasionally your physician must suggest institutionalization. You should abide by his decision because the child will benefit immensely from it. Most state institutions today are comfortable and provide excellent vocational and other education courses. Private institutions vary a great deal in their quality. Your neurologist will know best.

Is mental retardation dangerous?

The only dangerous types are the severely retarded, regardless of the cause, and the progressive types, which are few. People with these types of retardation often die of self-mutilation or accidents rather than spontaneous disease. With good diet and rest and the interest of others, however, retarded people can live to a ripe old age and many have a productive life.

What can I do to prevent it?

Avoid drugs and disease during pregnancy. Have an obstetrician deliver your baby, especially if you are prone to complications. Have a pediatrician take care of the baby immediately after birth. Other cases can be prevented by genetic counseling; your neurologist can advise you whether you should have children or not on the basis of your family background.

Multiple Sclerosis

What is multiple sclerosis?

This is a disease of the nervous system affecting young adults, which usually comes in repeated attacks but contrary to popular belief only occasionally cripples the victim.

What causes it?

The exact cause is unknown; however it is believed that the body produces antibodies against its own tissues, just as in rheumatic fever (page 227). In this case the antibodies attack the nerve tissue. It is similar to a "rash" of the nervous system.

What are the symptoms and signs of it?

The most common symptoms are blind spots in the eye, paralysis, numbness or tingling of the hands and/or feet, and difficulty walking. There may be dizziness, ringing in the ear, and double vision as well. Usually these symptoms come and go, lasting three to six weeks at a time, but their intensity may vary from day to day. Occasionally there is either incontinence or difficulty voiding. The attacks may be from a month to ten years apart. Some people have only one attack in their lives. There are no fever, chills or other constitutional symptoms.

What can I do about multiple sclerosis?

The condition will often clear up with bed rest and a low-fat diet. Severe cases require cortisone (page 305) or special injections of pituitary hormone (ACTH). Hospitalization is not usually necessary, as the diagnostic tests (including a spinal tap) can be done in a doctor's office.

Is it dangerous?

As stated above, very few people are crippled by this disease. Out of more than two hundred patients with multiple sclerosis in my practice, only one needs a wheel chair and none are blind.

What can I do to prevent it?

I know of nothing to prevent the initial attack for sure. However, to prevent subsequent attacks there's a lot you can do. I put all my patients on a low-fat diet with a minimum of milk and milk products. Then I prescribe calcium tablets with meals. A tranquilizer called Miltown seems to help this disease in my experience. Vitamin E and multivitamin tablets are also prescribed. You should avoid fatigue. Spinal anesthesia and vaccinations may precipitate an attack, so I don't allow them unless absolutely necessary.

Narcotic Addiction

What is narcotic addiction?

When we speak of addiction we usually mean physiologic or metabolic dependency on a drug. Most addiction of this type is addiction to narcotics, such as morphine or heroin or alcohol (see page 107). There are more than sixty thousand narcotic addicts in this country. Barbiturates and sedatives are another group of physiologically addicting drugs. Most dependency on barbiturates and other sedatives is psychological, however. Psychological addiction is simply a bad habit, and withdrawal of the drug rarely causes noticeable physical reactions. Cigarettes, coffee, and marihuana fall into this category also. LSD (lysergic acid diethylamide) doesn't cause physiologic addiction, but the hallucinatory trip is habit-forming.

What causes it?

Most people who become addicted or habituated have a significant psychiatric disorder, such as a neurosis (emotional disease) or a psychosis (mental disease). Social background is a predisposing factor; a large number of addicts are Negroes and Puerto Ricans from "ghetto" environments. Today the social pressures are also great among white, middle-class young people to try various illegally procured drugs. It is estimated that ninety percent of senior high school students have taken "speed" (Dexedrine) or marihuana.

What are the symptoms and signs of narcotic addiction?

Unless one is observed just after a "fix" or in the withdrawal state very few symptoms may be noted. There are constricted pupils in morphine or heroin addicts and dilated pupils in barbiturate or Demerol addicts. Heroin and morphine addicts may have injection marks on their arms and thighs. The administration of Nalline, a relative of morphine, will cause a withdrawal reaction in a narcotic addict. During abstinence from drugs the patient exhibits yawning, perspiration, tearing, and insomnia. There are often hot and cold flushes, generalized aches, and nausea and vomiting. Just after a "fix" there is a euphoria (feeling of well-being) so that the patient experiences extreme happiness, giddiness and occasional hallucinations. Withdrawal of barbiturates may induce nervousness, convulsions and coma.

What can I do about it?

See your doctor. He will hospitalize you, either locally or in an institution especially designed for this purpose. There you will withdraw under supervision, probably with the administration of methadone in gradually diminishing doses. Psychotherapy should be instituted in all cases. Unfortunately, only ten percent of addicts can be rehabilitated.

Is it dangerous?

It certainly is. Repeated doses of narcotics and sedatives create body tolerance (the need for larger doses each time to achieve the same effect). Since the drugs must often be obtained illegally, the high price causes people to steal. When they can't get the money, the "pusher" will often give them an overdose. Accidental overdoses are not uncommon. Occasional addicts die from tetanus (lockjaw) originating at a dirty injection site.

What can I do to prevent it?

Don't take narcotics, barbiturates, amphetamines or other addicting drugs except under a doctor's supervision. Narcotics should never be taken unless you have genuine pain in the first place. Don't associate with people who use any kind of drugs just for kicks. If you have a tendency to depend on any kind of drug (including aspirin) get psychiatric treatment. If you have chronic anxiety or depression you must get treatment also.

Nervous Breakdown

What is a nervous breakdown?

A nervous breakdown is a common lay term that usually means a severe emotional or mental illness requiring either care by a psychiatrist or a family doctor, or actual institutionalization, either in a local hospital or a mental hospital. This term has become so common that someone has even written a song called "I'm Having My Nineteenth Nervous Breakdown." If we use the milder definition of this term, meaning an emotional disturbance requiring treatment by a doctor, then at least eight out of ten people in the United States will suffer this at one time in their lives. The emotional disturbance may merely be a period of maladjustment to some problems at home, at work or with in-laws, etc. Then again, it may mean a more severe mental disturbance, such as depression from the change of life, a severe anxiety neurosis, or a psychosis, which would indicate a severe mental breakdown. I would say the term is usually used to imply that a person has actually had a psychotic breakdown, which means he had to receive treatment for months and sometimes up to two years. Certainly the term should not be one to be ashamed of because it is so common for Americans to have this. Particularly important to note is that suicide may result from a nervous breakdown. As an indication of how common a nervous breakdown must be, suicide is listed as the eighth cause of death in America.

Parkinson's Disease

What is Parkinson's disease?

Parkinson's disease is a disease of the nervous system of gradual onset, sometimes known as "shaking palsy" because it is associated with shaking.

What causes it?

No one knows the exact cause of idiopathic Parkinson's disease. A few cases are due to previous encephalitis, such as probably occurred during the "flu" epidemic of 1918, and another small group of cases may be due to hardening of the arteries. Some tranquilizers can cause similar symptoms.

What are the symptoms and signs of it?

The classical signs of Parkinson's are tremor and rigidity. This may be located on one, two, or all four extremities. The tremor is a shaking of the wrists, head and foot or legs. The rigidity makes it hard to move. Another symptom is inanition or lack of spontaneous movement (other than tremor) and initiative. Patients have expressionless face, a monotonous voice and walk bent forward with their arms at their sides. They do not have headaches or convulsions. There is no deterioration of intellect or memory.

What can I do about it?

You can do daily exercises to keep muscles from becoming too rigid, and stop worrying about it. Most cases are very slow in progression and some are arrested spontaneously. Your doctor has several drugs to stop the tremor and rigidity. Recently a large group of patients have responded well to L-dopa, an enzyme that seems to affect the brain somehow. Those patients who don't respond to medical treatment can have chemopallidectomy or chemothalamectomy. In this procedure, alcohol or some other substance is injected into the portion of the brain that contributes to the rigidity of Parkinsonism.

Is it dangerous?

It only becomes a threat to life after many years and then only if you give in to it.

What can I do to prevent it?

Nothing except avoid influenza.

Peptic Ulcer

What is peptic ulcer?

A peptic ulcer is an ulceration of the lining of either the stomach or the duodenum. Many of you have seen a break in the skin either from a cut or from an abrasion. Most of these heal without anything. But if the edges of the skin are separated by very much distance a chronic ulceration of the skin may develop. An ulcer in the stomach or duodenum (the first portion of the intestine) is similar to that. That is, there is a break in the lining of either of these two organs that does not heal very rapidly and therefore there is chronic festering of that area. If left untouched by a doctor or surgeon it may heal over a period of six to eight weeks, but the main reason that ulcers in the stomach and duodenum do not heal very rapidly is because of the constant irritation by acid and the enzymes (such as pepsin) secreted by the stomach and duodenum. Ulcers are very common in people between the ages of twenty and forty but they may occur at any age. They have occurred in two- or three-year-old infants and in older people in their eighties. Men seem to be more likely to have an ulcer than women. The reason for this is not known.

What causes a peptic ulcer?

I just stated that a peptic ulcer is caused by constant acidity and enzymes that are present in the stomach and duodenum. What increases the acidity? The emotional state of a person. Thus a person who is under chronic anxiety or has a lot of suppressed anger may have increased output of acid into the stomach and duodenum and at times this may break down the lining of the stomach and produce an ulcer. Sometimes these ulcers occur after acute stress in a person's life such as a sudden loss of a loved one or an automobile accident. More often, however, it is due to chronic stress, such as difficulties on the job or difficulties in a marriage. Ulcers may also occur in the esophagus or the jejunum (the lower portion of the intestinal tract) but these are much less frequent. Certain other types of body conditions may produce an ulcer, such as a tumor in the pancreas or even a brain tumor, but these are extremely rare.

What are the symptoms and signs of an ulcer?

Patients who have peptic ulcers usually complain of burning pain in their stomach or on the right side of their abdomen, usually immediately after a meal (as in the case of stomach ulcers) or one to two hours after meals (as in duodenal ulcers). This pain may go through to the back and there may be some burping and occasionally nausea and vomiting. If the ulcer gets deep enough it may bleed, so that a person may notice black stools. Sometimes the ulcers perforate, and then the patient is seized with acute pain all over his abdomen but particularly in the upper portion, and his abdomen becomes stiff. He may even go into shock. The pain frequently is relieved by taking Pepto-Bismol or some other antacid or by eating.

What can I do about an ulcer?

The most important things are proper medical supervision, a proper diet, and specific drugs, such as tranquilizers and an antispasmodic drug such as Pro-Banthine or its derivatives, which will relax the intestine and decrease the amount of acid that is secreted. The diets prescribed by doctors are usually based on frequent feedings of bland foods or milk so that the acid can be continually neutralized in the stomach and duodenum and the ulcer will have a better chance to heal. A very important part of treating the ulcer is to get the person on bed rest; sometimes it is better to do this in the hospital, where the meals can be brought to the patient and the patient can be completely relaxed, out of the environment of his home, where there may be wrangling children, etc. If this form of treatment (called medical treatment) is unsuccessful, then a surgeon must be called and one of the different types of gastrectomy (removing a portion of the stomach) is usually recommended. These operations are not serious when performed by a competent surgeon. The only problem with them is that you may develop an ulcer even after having had surgery. This is usually not the case. As I have stated above many of the ulcers may heal after six to eight weeks without any treatment, but it is much better to have supervision by the doctor so that the ulcer will heal without complications.

Is an ulcer dangerous?

An ulcer is in most cases not a dangerous condition, but if it is allowed to persist it may bleed and the patient may require several transfusions before he can recover. It may even rupture. This requires a different type of operation for sewing up the hole made by the ulcer.

How can I keep from getting an ulcer?

The best way is to have regular meals, regular sleep, good exercise, and a proper diet without using too much aspirin or coffee. Do not drink too heavily and refrain from smoking. Also, it would help to straighten out any emotional problems you may have in your life. Of course, this cannot always be accomplished easily.

Phlebitis

What is phlebitis?

Phlebitis is an inflammation of a vein, which usually occurs in the lower legs but may occur in any vein in the body. Since there is usually clotting of the blood in the area where the vein is inflamed, in medical circles this is referred to as thrombophlebitis.

What causes phlebitis?

Phlebitis is usually caused by an obstruction of the blood going through the veins. The blood fails to move very rapidly back to the heart in people with dilated veins such as varicose veins. It may occur in healthy people who do not move their legs enough and who usually sit at their jobs. Of course an inflammation of the veins may also occur if there is adjacent inflammation of the skin due to any type of infection whether it be bacterial, fungal or viral. Women who have just delivered their babies and have a very congested uterus may have thrombophlebitis in the pelvis. People who have hemorrhoids may develop thrombophlebitis in the hemorrhoidal veins as well as in the veins of the pelvis. People with heart disease, particularly with congestive heart failure, have a greater incidence of phlebitis. People who have too much blood in their veins, as in polycythemia, also have a greater incidence of phlebitis.

What are the signs of phlebitis?

If the phlebitis is acute there may be only stiffness in the calf or a little bit of pressure and slight pain in the area of the vein involved. The skin gets red around the vein and is very tender. There may be swelling of the legs with fluid below the area of inflammation of the vein. Sometimes, however, these symptoms do not bother the victim and the first sign of phlebitis is acute chest pain caused by the breaking off of a clot and its passage to the lung. This is a pulmonary embolism. This is why we want patients to get to the doctor at the first sign of phlebitis to prevent this complication.

What can I do about it?

The most important thing to do with phlebitis is to get your leg elevated and put warm soaks over the area of inflammation. This should be done with the supervision of a physician. If the phlebitis is superficial, that is, in the superficial veins of the leg, it may require nothing more than heat, elevation of the leg and bed rest. However, if it is in the deep veins, then your blood must be thinned so that the clot will not extend further up the leg and eventually break off and go to the heart and lungs. In addition, there are certain drugs that reduce the inflammation in the vein, such as Butazolidin and sometimes antibiotics. If the phlebitis leads to frequent embolisms in the lung, then it might be necessary to tie off the vein in question or to tie off the vena cava, which is the large vein leading from both legs into the heart.

Is it dangerous?

I think we have already answered this question above. This is very dangerous if it involves the deep veins of the leg, because the piece of clot can break off and go to the lung. Of course, in that case it will be signalled by swelling of the legs and pain in the calf.

What will happen if I don't do anything about it?

Ninety percent of the cases will clear up on their own even if you don't do anything, but if you have some associated disease such as a heart condition that is contributing to the phlebitis it is less likely that it will clear up on its own.

How can I prevent myself from getting phlebitis?

Good skin hygiene is very important; cutting out smoking will help prevent you from having phlebitis. In addition, if you have had frequent attacks of phlebitis then you should be on an anticoagulant continuously.

Pinkeye

What is pinkeye?

Pinkeye is usually an inflammation of the eye. In medical circles this is referred to as the acute red eye. An inflammation of the eye may be due to *conjunctivitis,* which affects the outer layer of the eye. It could be due to *iritis,* which affects the iris and the deep layer of the eye. It can be due to *scleritis,* which is due to inflammation of the whites of the eyes, or the red eye can be caused by glaucoma (see page 167).

The red eye can also be due to a foreign body in the eye, particularly if it is on the cornea. Occasionally people wake up with a hemorrhage of the eye, but this is usually nothing to worry about and clears up on its own. The hemorrhage is sometimes caused by coughing spells, which cause one of the small vessels in the conjunctiva to rupture. Inflammation of the conjunctiva is pretty common. Glaucoma is also common; however, iritis (inflamation of the iris) is much less frequent.

What is the cause of pinkeye?

We stated some of the causes above. *Conjunctivitis* is usually caused by a virus or bacteria. One of the common viruses is trachoma, which occurs in African countries, but the Koch-Weeks bacillus is a common cause of pinkeye in this country. The most frequent bacteria causing conjunctivitis are streptococcus, pneumococcus and gonococcus. Measles may cause a mild conjunctivitis, as well. The other causes of pinkeye mentioned above are foreign bodies, glaucoma and iritis. Iritis is usually caused by an allergic reaction in the body. It can also be caused by sarcoidosis or tuberculosis.

What are the symptoms and signs of pinkeye?

The signs of pinkeye are inflammation and reddening of the eye. There is pus in the eye and the person wakes up with a lot of "chicken feed" (dried pus) in the eye if it is due to an infection of the conjunctiva. If the condition is due to glaucoma or iritis there is usually not much of a discharge from the eye. The eye will itch if it is an allergic type of conjunctivitis. (It may also itch in any other type of conjunctivitis.) When there is glaucoma the symptoms that are mentioned in the section on glaucoma (page 167) will be experienced.

What can I do about pinkeye?

Of course, any problem with the eye should be seen immediately by a physician. There should be no delay, because a red eye may be something very serious. Treatment of conjunctivitis usually involves putting antibiotic drops in the eyes. With glaucoma you use the combination of drops and drugs given systemically mentioned in the pages on glaucoma. A foreign body must be removed immediately to prevent ulceration and loss of sight. Eye washes are a great help in conjunctivitis and will wipe it out in many cases, but this should only be done under the supervision of your physician.

Is an inflammation of the eye dangerous?

Yes! It will lead to loss of sight if it is not taken care of immediately in cases of glaucoma, iritis, and a foreign body.

What will happen if I don't do anything about it?

As I stated above you may lose your sight.

How can I prevent myself from getting it?

Since conjunctivitis is often transmitted in the large swimming pools we have today you can avoid swimming there. Also, avoid exposure to other people who have conjunctivitis. If you have a family history of glaucoma get frequent checks of your eyeball tension by your ophthalmologist.

Pneumonia

What is pneumonia?

Pneumonia is an infection of the lung, usually by a bacteria or a virus but occasionally by parasites and fungi. Pneumonia is one of the most common causes of death in this country, despite the fact that the incidence has been markedly reduced by the introduction of antibiotics such as penicillin.

What is the cause of pneumonia?

Pneumonia has many causes as mentioned above. They include viruses, bacteria, fungi, and parasites. However, the most common form of pneumonia is pneumococcal pneumonia. This is caused by the pneumococcus bacteria transmitted from one person to another through the air we breathe. The pneumococcus may be found in many healthy people's noses and throats. Another bacteria that commonly causes pneumonia, particularly in older people and people suffering from other severe diseases, is the staphylococcus bacteria. There are numerous other bacteria that may cause pneumonia. Influenza is a virus that may cause severe pneumonia at times, although more commonly it simply causes a bronchitis.

What are the symptoms and signs of pneumonia?

As most lay people well know, the most common symptom of pneumonia is a severe cough. This is usually accompanied by a fever, chills, and sweats, along with fatigue, weakness and loss of appetite. The cough is usually productive of a yellowish sputum but this may be rusty, as in the case of pneumococcal pneumonia, or there may be some frank blood in the sputum. When the pneumonia is severe it will cause severe shortness of breath. The person looks pale and may even be cyanotic, or blue.

What can I do about it?

Most people do not know that they have pneumonia until they go to a doctor and have him check them. At the first sign of fever with a cough productive of yellowish sputum, you should see your physician. He will be able to take a chest x-ray and examine your sputum and determine if you have any of the common causes of pneumonia. Once the diagnosis is made he will put you on appropriate therapy. This includes bed rest, a good expectorant, a humidifier, a bronchodilator drug, and—most important of all—antibotics such as penicillin. Fortunately, today we have many more antibiotics to combat pneumonia, and it is very rare for a bacteria to be resistant to all of these drugs. However, viral pneumonia still remains resistant to many drugs, and it takes two weeks to a month of bed rest to get rid of it.

Is it dangerous?

No. Pneumonia is not a dangerous disease today because of the tremendous antibiotics that we have. However, if you allow it to persist without treatment it can cause death. Pneumonia may be the final blow to some of our older people simply because they have such a run-down condition, or because of the aging process they are unable to combat any disease. That is why pneumonia is blamed as the cause of death so frequently in our country despite our excellent therapy for it.

What can I do to prevent pneumonia?

The best thing to do is to stay away from people who have pneumonia. However, if you must be exposed to them be sure you wear a mask over your face. In addition to that, keeping the proper diet, exercise and rest are very important in preventing yourself from getting pneumonia. If you have emphysema or asthma or other pulmonary diseases that predispose to pneumonia, then it may be wise for you to take an antibiotic. In addition it might be wise to get a flu vaccine at least every three months during the winter, since influenza predisposes one to pneumonia so often. People who live in crowded conditions, as in military barracks or in dormitories, are more prone to get pneumonia. This type of living quarters should be abandoned. In the hospital we isolate patients with pneumonia so that they will not affect others.

Prostate Trouble

What is prostate trouble?

Men who say they have "prostate trouble" usually mean they have trouble urinating because of an enlarged or inflamed prostate gland. The prostate gland is about the size of a walnut and is located at the mouth of a man's bladder. It secretes a fluid that lubricates the urethra (urinary passage) and creates a nourishing medium for the sperm when they pass.

What causes it?

Inflammation of the prostate gland can be caused by numerous bacteria and occasional viruses. Many cases are due to the venereal disease gonorrhea. Too much or too little intercourse may make one more susceptible to it. Enlargement of the prostate gland may be due to a cancer but more commonly to a simple, nonmalignant hypertrophy of the gland.

What are the symptoms of it?

As stated above, the most common symptom is difficulty urinating. You may have to stand awhile in front of the toilet before you can start the urine stream, or the stream may be interrupted in the middle. The stream is usually weak and there is frequently a drip at the end so that you feel is if you want to urinate more. This is because three or more ounces of urine may still be in the bladder. If there is infection the urine will burn as you void and you may have chills and fever. Also there will be a yellow or white discharge.

What can I do about it?

See your physician at once. He will do a rectal examination of the prostate gland and examine and culture your discharge and urine. He may catheterize you to see how much urine is left in your bladder after you void. If he diagnoses an inflamed prostate he will give you an antibiotic and massage your prostate weekly. If he diagnoses an enlarged or cancerous prostate he will advise an operation. Frequently you can be operated on without an incision by the doctor's passing an instrument called the cystoscope up the urinary passage and cauterizing or cutting pieces of the prostate away so that it won't obstruct the bladder. If you have cancer or if the gland is too large, he can't do it this way and you must have an abdominal incision or one near your rectum.

Is it dangerous?

Yes. If you don't get treatment infection will spread to the bladder and kidneys, or your kidneys will become blocked and destroyed and you will die of uremic poisoning.

What can I do to prevent it?

Avoid alcohol and cigarettes. Also avoid too much intercourse or abstaining. If you are single don't masturbate too often. Don't hold your water too long while traveling. Go to a service station or park alongside the road and go. Don't engage in intercourse with strange women, as they may have a venereal disease.

Psoriasis

What is psoriasis?

Psoriasis is a scaly eruption of the skin.

What causes it?

The exact cause is unknown but many cases are hereditary.

What are the symptoms and signs of it?

The scaly eruption and thickening of the skin does not usually itch and will bleed easily if you scratch it. It is located most commonly on the elbows, knees and feet but may occur anywhere.

What can I do about it?

Some excellent salves, such as Tegrin, can be purchased at the drug store without a prescription. A low-protein diet that is low in meat and eggs may help. If these measures don't work see your doctor. He has a variety of ointments, including cortisone preparations, that will help. Lipotriad, a type of vitamin preparation, may help.

Is it dangerous?

No. You will never die of it and its only harm is cosmetic and psychological.

What can I do to prevent it?

Nothing.

Rheumatic Fever

What is rheumatic fever?

Rheumatic fever is a febrile (marked by fever) disease affecting chiefly the joints, heart, skin and nervous system.

What causes it?

Almost all cases of rheumatic fever are preceded by a "strep" throat. It is believed that our blood produces antibodies against the streptococcus bacteria and its toxins that are also capable of attacking our own tissues, such as the heart and joints. Indeed, these antibodies can be found in the blood of people with rheumatic fever.

What are the symptoms and signs of it?

There are fever and chills; swollen, tender joints, particularly the knees and ankles; and heart murmurs in most cases. However, there may be a rash and/or St. Vitus dance (unusual, purposeless movements of the arms, legs and head). A sore throat with white patches on the tonsils will often be present. In some cases there is only a fever.

What can I do about it?

See your doctor at once. He will put you in the hospital for diagnostic tests and give you penicillin to cure the "strep" throat and aspirin in the proper dose to stop the disease. In some cases cortisone will be necessary. Bed rest for six weeks to three months will also be prescribed.

Is it dangerous?

Yes, left untreated you may develop heart congestion and die. Even when properly treated the disease may scar the valves of the heart and cause heart failure in later years.

What can I do to prevent it?

Get a well-balanced diet and eight hours of sleep a night. Avoid strep throat infections. People with enlarged tonsils should have them removed. Patients who have had rheumatic fever once should take penicillin daily for years later.

Shingles

What are shingles?

Shingles are a blistering rash of the skin usually in a specific area on one or the other side of the body.

What causes it?

A virus called herpes zoster causes shingles. Herpes zoster virus is a relative of, if not identical, with chicken pox virus. This virus affects the skin and the nerve roots.

What are the symptoms and signs of shingles?

Of course we have mentioned the rash, which usually consists of several half-inch blisters with water underneath. This gradually scabs over. This rash occurs on either one side or the other of the body in a specific area. Usually it occurs in a band of skin supplied by one or two nerves. In addition, since the virus affects the nerve root it causes severe pain. This pain may occur before the breaking out, with it, or afterwards for as long as six months to a year. The pain is very severe and will often keep a person awake during the night and interfere with his work. There is not usually any fever or any other constitutional symptom. But if the shingles are the result of some blood disease, then of course there will be symptoms from this blood disease.

What can I do about shingles?

Actually very little specifically can be done to kill the virus that causes shingles. The pain can be restricted by injections of a proteolytic substance and also by various creams applied to the blisters. Cortisone is sometimes used, but doctors are divided on their opinion as to whether this should be used or not. Various pain medicines have been applied with success. Your doctor will give you something in the form of a narcotic or other analgesic to kill the pain.

What will happen if I don't do anything about it?

If you don't do anything about it it will probably clear up on its own. It's usually nothing to worry about. There is one exception. If it hits the eyes, you will want an ophthalmologist to take care of you to prevent any serious effect upon your vision.

How can I prevent myself from getting it?

The best way is to keep from getting chicken pox as a kid, because there is so much evidence that the virus that causes shingles is the same as chicken pox. Adults who have not had chicken pox do not usually develop shingles. Instead they develop chicken pox when they are exposed to the virus.

Sinus Trouble

What is sinus trouble?

Sinus trouble, or sinusitis, usually means inflammation of the sinuses. This may be chronic or acute. Sinuses are usually inflammed during a common cold and occasionally they are blocked off by the common cold. Usually you have eight sinus cavities. These are the frontal sinuses, the maxillary sinuses, the sphenoid sinuses and the ethmoid sinuses, two of each. They are little pockets with a very small opening and they are usually lined with nasal mucosa. Since these openings pass into the nasal passages they can easily be blocked off by a cold. When they are blocked one of two things may occur: there may be a vacuum created in the sinus because the air is gradually absorbed and with the hole in the sinus blocked no more air can get in; or, there may be enough bacteria in the sinus to cause an infection, because with no drainage pus and mucus can accumulate in the blocked sinus.

What is the cause of sinusitis?

Sinusitis can be caused by the common cold, an allergy, or by other chronic inflammatory conditions of the nose. Too much smoking can cause inflammation of the nasal mucosa and subsequent blocking of small holes that lead from the sinuses into the nose. Occasionally the sinuses are involved by a polyp or a tumor. When a sinus is blocked and pus accumulates in it we usually consider this an acute sinusitis. Chronic sinusitis is not uncommon; it is usually a milder inflammation of the lining of the sinuses and does not necessarily involve a blocking of the small holes that lead from the sinuses into the nose.

What are the symptoms of sinusitis?

Usually the most common symptom is headache. This may be frontal or occipital (at the back of the head) or it may be a pain over the cheeks. There is also tenderness over the involved sinuses! Your doctor will look into your nose and will look for discharges from the sinus openings. He will also transilluminate the sinuses with light in a dark room. Often, however, x-rays are necessary to observe all eight sinus cavities for pus accumulations or for tumors.

What can I do about it?

If you have a mild inflammation of the sinuses without the accumulation of pus all you need are nasal decongestants, taken by drops, spray, or orally—such as Dristan advertised on television. Your doctor has a drug called Ornade which is stronger than Dristan. Your doctor may want to drain the sinuses himself by applying nasal decongestants directly to the openings of the sinuses. But if you have an accumulation in one of the sinus cavities, then it is necessary to pass a catheter into the sinuses and wash them out. This can be easily performed in the physician's office. Patients who have had chronic sinusitis for a long period of time may have to have the diseased mucosal lining removed and a larger hole between the sinuses and nose created. This might be performed by an E.N.T. (ear, nose, and throat) specialist.

What will happen if I don't do anything about it?

Usually very little because the sinuses usually clear up and infection passes, but you will suffer a great deal of discomfort if you do not get treatment immediately. Rarely the sinus infection may get into your blood stream and cause a generalized infection.

Smoking

Smoking is by far one of the most hazardous things that a man does to damage his health. We are our own worst enemy when it comes to our health. We smoke, we eat too much, we drink, we don't get enough exercise and we allow ourselves to get involved in tension- and depression-producing situations. All of these together account for the major causes of death, which as you know are cancer, heart disease, and stroke. Smoking contributes directly and indirectly to diseases of the blood vessels, of the heart, of the brain, and to cancer. It also has been implicated in automobile accidents and other accidents, particularly fires. So it should not be hard to say that smoking presents the greatest danger to health in our time. It is more dangerous than tuberculosis, pneumonia, and other diseases.

How does smoking contribute to diseases of the body?

In cigarettes and cigars there is a great deal of nicotine. Nicotine constricts the blood vessels to the heart, causing a heart attack. It may constrict the blood vessels to the brain, causing a stroke! It may constrict the blood vessels to the lower legs, causing ulcers in the legs and occlusions of the arteries to the legs necessitating amputation of the leg. It constricts the blood vessels to the lungs, making it difficult for the blood to pass through the lungs to get oxygenated. Nicotine also constricts the small muscles in the bronchial tubes. In this way, it obstructs the breathing and may lead to the condition called pulmonary emphysema, in which air cannot get out of the lungs once it gets in.

The tar in the tobacco causes cancer of the lungs and it may also be a cause of cancer in the bladder and other areas of the body. Nicotine or some other factor in tobacco may increase the cholesterol in the blood and lead to increased fat and hardening of the arteries.

How much smoking a person can do without getting cancer, heart disease or stroke is hard to say. A pack or more a day is definitely implicated in lung cancer, heart disease and stroke. If one limits himself to five or six cigarettes a day it is unlikely that he will ever get any of these diseases from smoking itself. But how many people can do this?

What can I do about it?

You can stop smoking! It is very difficult for a person to cut down to five or six cigarettes a day. Most people do not have the willpower to do this. They must stop altogether. Your physician will prescribe a tranquilizer while you are doing this. This will help relieve some of the tension. You may attend a smoking clinic where other smokers are gathered together to try to help each other quit. This form of psychotherapy is very valuable but it does not work with everybody. A very good substitute for smoking is chewing gum. There are drugs on the market such as Nicoban (a form of alphalobeline) that may substitute for the nicotine craving of many heavy smokers, but this does not always work. Getting proper religious guidance may help. Some people have been able to use a belief in God and a desire to live a clean life as a means of destroying their desire for cigarettes. I would rather see you overeat or drink too much alcohol than smoke cigarettes, because it is so damaging to your health. Naturally, I would not want you to do any of these three if you could avoid it, but if eating or drinking is the only way you can keep from smoking then do it!

One of the reasons Americans smoke too much is that they have too much free time. Another reason is that they live a fast-moving life with great tension at work. With over nine million divorces since 1945 it is understandable that we are living in a tension-producing society. This is definitely going to increase the amount of smoking we do. If we could eliminate the factors that cause tension we could eliminate the need to smoke. The best way to prevent smoking is proper education of the public, particularly children and teenagers before they start smoking. During youth, smoking seems to be a desirable thing to do to impress others. People who are involved in sports, music and other hobbies have less tendency to smoke because these hobbies relieve a lot of tension. There are other ways of reducing the desire to smoke that would take pages and pages to discuss.

Strokes

What is a stroke?

To most laymen a stroke is a blood clot in the brain. Actually, a stroke is the damage to a section of the brain due to loss of its blood supply by occlusion or hemorrhage of one of the major arteries or its branches to the brain. If the vessel that supplies the damaged area of the brain is merely occluded for a short period of time or partially occluded, then there may be complete recovery of the damaged tissue and the patient may suffer only temporary paralysis. If the vessel is completely occluded by a clot, fat or calcium, then the area in question may not make a complete recovery. Each year over a half million people in the United States suffer from a stroke. Ninety percent of these people have a stroke due to a clot or obstruction of the vessel. The other ten percent have a hemorrhage from the vessel into the surrounding brain tissue.

What is the cause of a stroke?

As said above the main cause of a stroke is a clot occluding one of the cerebral vessels or a hemorrhage into the brain. The most common cause of the obstruction is arteriosclerotic disease of the blood vessels, the same condition that affects the walls of the coronary arteries supplying the heart. Usually deposits of cholesterol accumulate on these vessels over the years and the lumen (hollow center) of the vessels becomes gradually narrowed. If the lumen becomes so narrow that the blood becomes very sluggish going through it, the blood may clot before it gets through it.

The most common cause of hemorrhage, on the other hand, is hypertension. In this case the blood pressure in the circulation gets so high that it ruptures the blood vessels. Then the blood permeates into the surrounding brain, causing damage. Hemorrhages may result in younger people due to an inborn weakness in the walls of the blood vessels supplying the brain. These are called aneurysms, and they cause a bulging of the artery almost as your automobile tire will bulge if there is a weakness in one area of it.

Sometimes the blood vessels are occluded by an embolism from somewhere else in the body, such as the heart. This embolism may be made up of calcium, fat, or air, or it could be a clot coming from the heart.

What are the symptoms and signs of a stroke?

Most of you are familiar with the paralysis that occurs with a stroke. It is usually one arm and one leg on the same side of the body. Many other types of symptoms may occur with a stroke. Often people faint or become very confused and weak. Sometimes a stroke may cause only numbness or tingling in one arm or one leg. It may affect only the speech. There can be difficulty walking and there may be loss of control of the bladder or bowels. Severe headaches can occur when there is a hemorrhage into the brain, and this may be associated with stiffness of the neck. The patient gradually lapses into a coma as the hemorrhages get larger. Usually a stroke does not cause a drop in the blood pressure as happens in the case of strokes in the heart or coronary occlusions, but occasionally a stroke does lower the blood pressure; and usually with a hemorrhage the blood pressure rises.

What can I do about a stroke?

The most important thing is to get immediate treatment by a doctor. Most patients with a stroke have to be admitted to a hospital for evaluation. It is important to determine whether the stroke was due to a hemorrhage or a thrombosis (clot). If it is due to a thrombosis it is important to put the patient on blood thinners in some cases and to give vasodilators to dilate the blood vessels. On the other hand if the stroke is due to a hemorrhage it is important to bring the blood pressure down so that further hemorrhaging will not occur. Sometimes the stroke is due to occlusion of the large vessels outside of the brain in the neck. Then a surgeon can be called in to remove the clot in the blood vessel or to install an artificial artery by-passing the clot so that the blood can continue to flow to the brain. Also it is important to determine whether the stroke was due to an embolism, or a piece of clot coming from the heart. Perhaps the heart was the first organ to be involved with a "stroke" (coronary occlusion), and then a piece of clot broke off from the inside of the heart and went to the brain.

There are actual stroke-care units in many hospitals in this country, analogous to coronary care units, with specialized nurses and other technical help to take care of the patient with a stroke. The patients are turned frequently and their limbs are exercised. They have a catheter placed in their bladder if necessary. Other forms of physiotherapy are applied. The patient requires a lot of rest to get over a stroke. Once it is determined how much of the function of an arm or leg or the speech is lost, trained specialists can be called in to help the patient regain as much control as possible of the areas that are disabled. It may require as much as three to six months of rehabilitation in a hospital to get the patient back to as full a recovery as possible.

Is a stroke dangerous?

If the stroke is just due to an occlusion of a blood vessel the patient may not suffer any threat to his life, but the damage to the brain may be severe enough to cause complete paralysis and he will be helpless. In many cases, however, the patient regains his full or at least partial use of the arm and leg or other areas involved and can assume a fairly normal life. A lot of these patients return to work and live a productive life.

What will happen if I don't do anything about a stroke?

If the stroke is due to a hemorrhage you will almost certainly die because the mortality rate is high. If the stroke is due to thrombosis, of course, you may continue to get more and more paralyzed and not only lose the use of one arm or one leg but maybe all four extremities. This is why you should consult your doctor immediately. If you have a wife who is a very attentive person she may be able to take care of you throughout the illness without hospitalization but she will need the supervision of your family doctor.

How can I prevent myself from having a stroke?

The prevention of a stroke is similar to the prevention of a heart attack. You should get plenty of rest, regular exercise, stop smoking, eat a well balanced diet, particularly one low in cholesterol, and you should have frequent checkups by your physician with blood tests for cholesterol and other fat. It is important to keep your blood pressure down, and if your physician discovers high blood pressure, be sure to take your medicine so that you do not get precipitous elevations that may cause a rupture of one of the arteries of the brain. If you have had a previous stroke your doctor may find it wise to keep you on a blood thinner to prevent you from having another one. This will depend on many factors including your blood pressure. If your blood pressure is high he may not want to put you on a blood thinner for fear the chance of blood leaking into the brain would be greater.

People who have experienced a little stroke with transient weakness in an arm or leg, or transient numbness and tingling in an arm or leg, or transient loss of speech should report to their physician about these so that he can treat them before they develop a permanent paralysis from a complete occlusion of a cerebral artery.

Tuberculosis

What is tuberculosis?

Tuberculosis is an infectious disease primarily of the lungs but sometimes affecting other organs of the body. Tuberculosis is a form of pneumonia. Tuberculosis is a very highly contagious disease and used to be one of the major causes of death and disability in this country. However, through proper hygiene, better living conditions and better treatment and diagnosis this disease has been to a large extent wiped out. While tuberculosis is still a problem in the crowded and poverty stricken areas of our country, if you are practicing medicine in the suburbs you may not see more than one case of tuberculosis a year.

What is the cause of tuberculosis?

Tuberculosis is caused by the tubercle bacillus, a bacteria. This bacteria infects human beings largely from personal contact or from breathing the air from an infected person. It can even be transmitted by kissing.

What are the symptoms and signs of tuberculosis?

Many patients with tuberculosis have no symptoms at all and they are only picked up by periodic chest examinations and tuberculin tests. However, when symptoms manifest there is often fever and night sweats, a chronic cough usually with yellowish sputum or blood, and loss of weight. There may be weakness, fatigue, and loss of appetite as well. Occasionally a person complains of glandular swelling in the neck or some other part of the body, but this is less likely. Sometimes tuberculosis causes symptoms in an organ other than the lung. In the kidney it may cause blood in the urine. In the brain a meningeal reaction occurs with headache, stiff neck and high fever.

What can I do about tuberculosis?

Fortunately, today very much can be done about tuberculosis. Your doctor has a variety of drugs, such as PAS (para-aminosalicyclic acid), isoniazid, streptomycin, and others, to combat tuberculosis. In addition there are several sanitariums around the country where one can go to get proper rest, nutrition, and climate so that recovery can be promoted. A very important part of your treatment is to avoid exposure to others. This is the main reason for putting people in sanitariums today. It used to be that many people with tuberculosis had a poor diet, lived in crowded areas, and had inadequate rest. This was the main reason for the sanitariums then. If you do not have tubercle bacilli in your sputum you may even be treated at home without hospitalization. However if you have small children at home it is wise to be hospitalized, regardless of whether there is tubercle bacilli found in your sputum or not. I have personally treated many patients at home, and they even continue to work. If the tubercle bacillus invades too much of the lung it may be necessary to do a lobectomy (remove a portion of the lung). This will be done by a thoracic surgeon. Older methods of treatment for tuberculosis, such as pneumothorax, have been pretty much outdated by the excellent therapy we have today.

Is tuberculosis dangerous?

It is no longer as dangerous as previously because of the drugs that we have and also the excellent surgical procedures. However, it must be mentioned that adequate nutrition and rest must be combined with these new drugs.

How can I prevent myself from getting tuberculosis?

The best thing to do is to stay away from people who have active tuberculosis. Next to that is good nutrition, adequate rest, and a job in a nonpolluted environment. Finally, if you smoke you should stop. It is very important to get a chest x-ray at least once a year and a tuberculin test periodically if you want to catch tuberculosis early. This is a very important part of prevention. The public health service has set up mass screening surveys for next to nothing in cost to you.

Varicose Veins

What are varicose veins?

Varicose veins are dilated veins usually seen in the lower legs but of course they may be seen in the arms and the abdomen as well. A hemorrhoid is actually a varicose vein, a dilated vein in the area of the rectum.

What causes varicose veins?

Usually varicose veins are caused by a combination of a hereditary predisposition to varicose veins (ordinarily a weakening in the walls of the veins due to something in the genetic makeup of the individual) and the long hours that an individual may spend on his feet during the day. Workers such as barbers, dentists or store clerks who have a hereditary predisposition to developing varicose veins are very likely to get them; because these people stand on their feet a long time, the walls of their veins are weakened by back pressure and then the valves in the veins give way so that the blood does not flow toward the heart as it normally should but backs up. Another cause of varicose veins is obstruction, either on the inside or extrinsic pressure on the outside of the vein obstructing the blood flow to the heart. You actually have hundreds of veins in each leg and only a few of them may be dilated and become varicose, but these cause such an ugly appearance that you naturally feel that all of your veins are dilated.

What are the symptoms and signs of varicose veins?

Of course varicose veins that are close to the surface are easily recognized by dilated areas of veins. Other signs, however, are small hemorrhages into the skin or even pain in the muscles from hemorrhages of the deep varicose veins. Occasionally the varicose veins form a clot inside, and this leads to phlebitis with red hot swelling over the vein. Another sign of varicose veins is simply swelling in the legs, particularly at the end of the day. If a person has had varicose veins for a long time, the skin of his lower legs may assume a freckled appearance and even be dark and grey if the varicose veins are obstructed by clots. Then varicose ulcers may develop in the legs. Itching of the legs is another symptom.

What can I do about varicose veins?

Fortunately there has been an excellent operation devised called ligation and stripping of these veins. This is performed by a surgeon who is very competent in this area.

The ligation and stripping can be as extensive as is necessary to clean up all the veins, but few surgeons take longer than two or three hours to perform this operation. It can go on for four to six hours if one expects to clean up every vein. This requires only about seven days in the hospital, but your period of convalescence may be longer. This is not a dangerous operation and if you think that your veins are very ugly and a surgeon agrees with you then I think you should go ahead and have it done. Another treatment that has been popular from time to time but at the present time is not too popular is injection of a sclerosing solution into the veins; the trouble with this procedure is that it has to be repeated frequently. Of course, ligation and stripping may also have to be done a second or a third time.

What will happen if I don't do anything about varicose veins?

If you don't have the operation performed, obviously you will just continue to have the poor cosmetic appearance in your legs for year after year. However, you can go head and wear ace bandages to keep the swelling down. Keep your legs propped up as frequently as possible when you are not walking. You may develop a clot in the legs (phlebitis) as mentioned above, and you also may develop ulcers in the lower legs, or even dermatitis.

How can I prevent varicose veins from developing?

Well, this is usually done by wearing ace bandages or elastic stockings all the time. Women should avoid becoming pregnant. Pregnancy definitely aggravates varicose veins because the head of the fetus obstructs the veins in the pelvis. Also, you can change your occupation from standing to one of sitting or one where you do a great deal of moving about.

Venereal Disease

What is venereal disease?

Venereal disease generally speaking is a disease transmitted from one sex to another by intercourse. Of course, with the rising homosexuality venereal diseases can be transmitted between members of the same sex. There are five basic venereal diseases. These are: gonorrhea, syphilis, chancroid, granuloma inguinale, and lymphogranuloma venereum. Gonorrhea and syphilis are the most common. Nine million living Americans have or have had syphilis at one time. In Pennsylvania in 1964 there were 14,205 cases of venereal disease reported. In 1971 we have been told the disease is rapidly on the increase. At the present time one million two hundred thousand Americans have untreated syphilis, and many of them do not know that they have it. There are probably about twenty-eight thousand syphilitic patients in the mental institutions of Pennsylvania alone.

What accounts for the tremendous rise in V.D.?

Probably the main reason is the increasing promiscuity in our society. Up until the penicillin era it was common sense not to have sexual relations before marriage and not to have extramarital relations. There was always a fear of this dread disease, which could not be cured until penicillin and sulfa came into existence. Now people no longer fear this disease. Also, the other main deterrent of sexual intercourse—the possibility of pregnancy—has been surmounted because of the birth control pills and other means of contraception.

Another reason that syphilis and gonorrhea are problems is because a lot of people don't know they have it, particularly women. Other people who have it aren't informed that there is treatment and do not bother to get it. Still other people are embarrassed to tell that they have it and will seek treatment only from a family doctor. In certain areas there is no family doctor that they can confide in. Let's take each of these types of V.D. and discuss them from a standpoint of symptoms and what you can do about them.

GONORRHEA

What are the symptoms and signs of gonorrhea?

Gonorrhea is a venereal disease caused by a bacteria called the gonococcus. Like other V.D. it is transmitted by intercourse. About three to seven days following intercourse the patient notices that he has burning on urination and a yellowish discharge from the penis or vagina. If this is allowed to continue both the male and female may have spread of the infection up the urinary tract. Most devastating to the female is the spread of the infection to the womb and the tubes. She may develop a severe salpingitis (inflammation of the tubes). Occasionally she develops severe abdominal pain and cramps along with a temperature. The male may have the infection spread up through the spermatic cord into the testicles and develop a severe swelling and inflammation of the testicle and epididymis, which are tubes adjacent to the testicles. Unfortunately, gonorrhea allowed to continue beyond the initial stage may spread into the blood stream and go to the heart or to the joints. Occasionally it is spread by the fingers from the urethra to the eyes. Your physician can easily make a diagnosis of gonorrhea by taking a smear from the vagina or the penis and looking at it under the microscope. Occasionally he can find the bug only by culturing it in special media. In the secondary stage it may be difficult to diagnose in this manner. Then almost invariably cultures and even a special type of serological blood test are necessary to diagnose this disease.

What can I do about gonorrhea?

Most cases of gonorrhea can be wiped out by one or two shots of penicillin. A few cases have been found to be resistant to this drug and require terramycin or one of the other antibiotics. When the disease progresses beyond the primary stage into the testicles or into the womb and the tubes, then the treatment must be continued for longer periods of time, and since in women secondary invaders sometimes develop, other antibiotics are necessary. If the disease has progressed to the heart or to the joints, then the treatment must also be for a longer period of time.

This disease could actually be wiped completely off the map if all people who had symptoms of a discharge from their penis or vagina would report immediately to their physician. It could also be done if everyone were to refrain from intercourse for a period of six months to a year and all those people with discharges were to report to their doctors. Another possible method would be to inoculate everybody over twelve, thirteen or fourteen years of age with penicillin; however, this would be difficult to do with people who are allergic to penicillin. It is unlikely that either of the latter two procedures would be followed, so the best thing is for people to report to their doctors as soon as they notice a discharge. They should also mention the names of any sexual contacts. It is easy to see that this is a dangerous disease if it is allowed to go untreated. It is a shame that women spread this disease to their children's eyes at birth because of their ignorance or their shame of admitting they might have this condition.

SYPHILIS

The symptoms of syphilis in the male are usually an ulcer around the penis and swelling of the glands in the groin. This is usually a painless ulcer which is called a *chancre*. There is very little discharge from it. If the disease is allowed to pursue its course without treatment, the ulcer will probably disappear, but in most cases syphilis has already invaded the blood by that time and will lead to systemic complications. The organism that causes syphilis is a motile spiral-shaped organism that can be easily seen under a dark-field microscope. In the female the development of the chancre is less likely to be noticed. Some of the chancres appear inside the vagina, and women frequently discover their condition only after the disease has invaded the blood stream. Then it is in the secondary stage. In the secondary stage both male and female develop a rash over their entire body, enlargement of the lymph nodes, occasionally enlargement of the spleen and liver, and other symptoms. There is a third stage of this disease almost similar to gonorrhea, where the syphilis involves the heart, particularly the large artery leading out of the heart called the aorta, and the nervous system, causing a person to become crippled or demented. If the mother passes the disease on to her child while it is in the womb, then the child develops a certain type of syphilis called congenital syphilis. Here the organism affects many organs of the body.

How do you diagnose it?

The doctor must take blood for a serology, which is always performed before marriages. You can take material from the active ulcer of the penis or the labia (vaginal lips) and look at this under a dark-field microscope. Once the disease has progressed to the brain a spinal tap may be necessary to find the spirochete or to perform a serology on the spinal fluid. Fortunately, today we have diagnostic tests that can give almost a hundred percent diagnosis.

What can I do about it?

Fortunately here is another venereal disease that can be treated effectively with penicillin. If it is caught in its primary stage it can be completely wiped out. In the third stage it is more difficult to treat, but eighty to ninety percent of people who have the third stage can be adequately treated with penicillin. The disease is communicable only in the primary and to a certain extent in the secondary stage. Therefore, it is important to treat people in the primary stage to prevent this condition from smoldering in the body. Here is another disease that could be wiped out by voluntary abstention from intercourse, but it is unlikely that people will ever do this. Mass inoculation by penicillin would be an extremely difficult undertaking, because it takes more than one shot to wipe out the third stage of syphilis, and a few of the patients in the third stage would not be cured. Also, those people who are allergic to penicillin could not receive the drug. However, if massive inoculation was performed most cases of primary syphilis could be eliminated and we could cut down on the rapid rate of spread of this illness.

OTHER VENEREAL DISEASES

Chancroid

Chancroid is another venereal disease that, like syphilis, produces an ulcer, but in this case it is usually a painful ulcer.

It appears about three to five days after exposure, and there is often a swelling in the groin, which is called a "bubo." Your doctor can make the diagnosis by taking a smear from the ulcer and culturing it. While this disease does not respond very well to penicillin, it responds extremely well to other antibiotic treatment that your doctor knows about.

Granuloma inguinale

This is an ulcerative skin disease that is caused by a bacteria. The symptoms of this disease are multiple small ulcers that appear one to twelve weeks after exposure on the penis or nearby. They also cause swelling of the glands in the groin. Here again the doctor makes a diagnosis by placing scrapings from the ulcer under the microscope. Like chancroid, the treatment of this disease is with antibiotics other than penicillin.

Lymphogranuloma venereum

This is a disease caused by a virus. The symptoms are a small red blister on the penis or around the vagina that develops about five to twelve days after exposure. There is enlargement of the lymph glands in the groin following this, and there may be enlargement of the liver and some constitutional symptoms such as fever or chills. In later stages there may be strictures of the rectum, making it difficult to move the bowels. The diagnosis is made by a skin test similar to the tuberculin test called the Frei test, but it can also be made on blood tests for serology. Unfortunately this disease is not as easy to treat as the other venereal diseases, but it usually responds to tetracycline.

In summary, the venereal diseases, particularly syphilis and gonorrhea, are on the increase because of increased promiscuity in our society, mostly among teenagers. Yet here are diseases that can be treated remarkably well. It is no longer tolerable for us to abide with diseases that spread so rapidly from one person to another. Massive public health measures should be taken to wipe them out. People should be educated so that they do not fear revealing their symptoms so much and will get early treatment. People should take the proper precautions when they have extramarital, premarital, and even marital relations when they are uncertain of their partner's fidelity or cleanliness.

Warts

What are warts?

A wart is a thickening or elevation of the skin or a polypoid growth on the skin, usually no more than one-half centimeter and most frequently about one to two millimeters in diameter. These are one of the most common skin diseases.

What causes warts?

Warts are caused by a virus. They are not a cancer as lots of people think. Yet it is because of the fact that we have discovered that warts are caused by a virus that scientists are looking into the possibilities that cancer is caused by viruses.

What are the symptoms and signs of a wart?

Warts can occur anywhere on the skin of the body, but the most common area is around the palms, soles, armpits and neck. Another common area is on the face. Occasionally warts even occur on the lips or the mucous membranes or in the vagina and rectum. Warts are usually painless. They do not exude any pus or other material. A lot of people peel them off but they can grow back because their roots are deep. However, there is one type of wart—the plantar wart—that is painful, because instead of the thickened material growing out on the skin surface, it grows into the subcutaneous tissues.

What can I do about a wart?

Warts can be removed by acid, such as trichloroacetic acid, or they can be cauterized. Your doctor may want to inject a sclerosing solution such as sodium morrhuate into the wart. Warts can be excised surgically but you must be sure you get the roots of the wart. Plantar warts are especially hard to treat. It is very difficult to excise the entire amount by surgery. Some physicians use x-ray treatment but only as a last resort. There have been other methods, such as witchcraft, which are said to be highly effective. But why do that when your doctor can have a hundred percent success if he uses medical methods?

Is a wart dangerous?

No!

What will happen if I don't do anything about it?

Most warts will continue to grow if you don't do anything about them but sometimes they spontaneously disappear after three to five years. The worst thing is that one wart may spread and produce other warts.

Whiplash Injury

What is a whiplash injury?

A whiplash injury is usually an acute extension and flexion of the neck that occurs when the body is thrown backwards by a blow from the rear. This usually occurs in an automobile accident when one car is hit from behind by another car. The neck is extended at first and thrown backwards and then the neck is flexed forward as a secondary reaction to the hyperextension. This injury may also occur in competitive sports such as football or in a fall down the steps, etc. This injury may cause tearing of the ligaments of the neck; it may cause rupture of the disc in the cervical spine; it may even lead to fracture of the spine at times. The muscles of the neck may suffer small or large hemorrhages into their substance. If the fracture or the rupture of the disc is big enough it may cause compression of the spinal cord with complete paralysis below the compression (paraplegia, quadraplegia).

What are the signs of a whiplash injury?

The patient usually gives a history of having had an automobile accident and usually has been hit from behind or the side. He suffers great pain in his neck and sometimes pain radiating down his arms. Occasionally he may have numbness in his head, hands or his feet. He may have severe headaches as well. Some patients are confused after an injury of this nature and they may be in emotional shock for several days or even months after. This may be witnessed by depression even to the point of crying, loss of sleep, and loss of appetite. However, pain in the neck radiating into the back of the head is the most common symptom.

What can I do about it?

Many people see their lawyer before they see their doctor, but it is wise to see your doctor first. He will perform x-rays of your skull and cervical spine to exclude the possibility of a fracture or a ruptured disc, and that, along with his clinical examination, can at least rule out the most hazardous complications of a whiplash injury. However, to eliminate your pain he must give you analgesics and muscular relaxants and often prescribe a collar to be worn both night and day for awhile. If this is ineffective you may require cervical traction and eventually evaluation for surgery. Sometimes plain x-rays of the neck do not pick up a herniated disc, and therefore a myelogram must be performed to rule this out. Of course, if a herniated disc is discovered then surgery would be advisable in most cases. The problem with most people that develop a whiplash is that they have a certain amount of arthritis due to the "calcium deposits" that develop in the cervical spine over the years. Severe hyperextension of the neck and subsequent flexion causes these calcium deposits to become symptomatic. It is often difficult for the doctor to determine how much of the patient's pain is due to preexisting cervical arthritis and how much is due to the automobile accident.

Is it dangerous to have whiplash injury?

In the vast majority of cases the whiplash injuries are not dangerous and they do not cause any serious complications.

What will happen if you don't do anything about it?

In most cases your pain, headache, numbness and tingling will go away in six months to a year. However I have found that people who seek the aid of a lawyer in getting adequate compensation for their injury seem to have symptoms much longer than those who don't. Sometimes it is better to suffer the moderate amount of pain one experiences with a whiplash injury under the care of a competent physician and try to settle the insurance claims without the aggravation of going to court. Your symptoms may clear up quicker. One of the worst problems in this country is the tremendous backlog of compensation cases. If people could get their claims settled immediately I feel they would return to work sooner and their symptoms would disappear much sooner.

DIAGNOSTIC TESTS

Biopsy

What is a biopsy?

A biopsy is the removal of a small portion of tissue from any organ of the body to be submitted for pathological examination under the microscope. A biopsy may be made up of skin, liver, lung, brain, and any other organ.

Why is a biopsy performed?

Most frequently a biopsy is performed to diagnose cancer of the organ from which the tissue is taken. However, a biopsy of the liver is frequently done to diagnose hepatitis or cirrhosis of the liver. A biopsy of the brain is performed occasionally to diagnose degenerative diseases of the brain. Frequently a biopsy is performed just prior to the removal of an organ. Thus the operation may be interrupted momentarily while the pathologist examines a small portion of the tissue for cancer, and if cancer is found then the whole organ is removed. This is a frequent procedure when a lump in the breast is operated on. If cancer is not found then the breast or other organ involved can be left untouched.

How is a biopsy performed?

Frequently a biopsy is performed with a special needle devised to remove a piece of tissue from the organ in question. Biopsies of the liver, lung, and even the kidney are performed in this fashion. However, almost as frequently the biopsy is performed by an incision into the organ under direct vision. This type of biopsy procedure is frequently performed in cancer of the prostate, stomach or testicles.

Is a biopsy dangerous?

No, a biopsy is rarely dangerous. There are a few organs in which a biopsy may cause spread of the cancer, but your doctor has the sense not to perform biopsies on these organs when cancer is likely.

Blood Test

What is a blood test?

Nowadays a blood test is not just one test. It usually involves taking a blood sample that can be used for several different tests. The analysis of blood for diseased states has become such an important part of medical science today that whole sections of the hospitals are devoted to laboratory facilities for testing blood for various substances. Thus we can test your blood for sugar or cholesterol (a very important fat in the blood). We can test your blood cells; and the quality and the number of these cells is very important in diseased states. We can test it for its coagulation. We can test it for the urine in the blood (blood urea nitrogen) and the uric acid in the blood (to diagnose gout). We can test the blood for calcium and other salts, to determine whether you have too much or too little of these chemicals. We can test the blood for various enzymes, which pour into the blood when various tissues in your body break down and are diseased. These are only a few of the tests. We can even test your blood for several types of hormones.

What happens when I get a blood test?

Usually you go to the doctor's office or the hospital and are seated in a chair with your arm resting on the chair; the technician will put a tourniquet on your upper arm, scrub your elbow area and palpate for a vein. When she finds the the vein then she will take a syringe with a needle on it and insert this into the vein and draw out five or ten cubic centimeters of blood or (between one-quarter and one-third of an ounce of blood). Today this amount of blood can be used for up to twenty different tests, so don't fear that because you have several blood tests to be done she will require a lot of blood. Actually, however, you could have a blood test every day for several weeks and still not be drained of all the blood that is necessary for your body function. Your body has a tremendous capacity to make new blood. Indeed many hospital patients have this blood test performed every day for months.

Is a blood test dangerous?

A blood test is no more dangerous than crossing the street. It is rare for the needle to cause an infection, and even if it does it will clear up without any trouble. With our new disposable needles it is very unlikely that you will ever get hepatitis or any other infections. There are a few people who develop a tremendous anxiety in anticipation of a needle, and some people even faint as a result of having a needle inserted into their body, but these people come out of the faint without any complications. Remember, you will not bleed to death from a small needle puncture! With the hundreds of thousands of people in this country having blood tests every day it is very unlikely that it is a dangerous procedure or these people would be complaining. Most people think that a blood test is only performed when you are getting married or to find out if you have a venereal disease. This is only one reason that a blood test is performed, as you can surmise from the above discussion.

Brain Wave Test

What is a brain wave test?

A brain wave test, or electroencephalogram, is the recording of the electrical discharges from your brain by means of an electroencephalogram machine, linked to your head by numerous tiny electrodes. The brain is made up of eight billion or more tiny cells, each with an electrical charge on it, and when a human being is thinking or moving his muscles, these little nerves are excited and give off an electrical charge. This charge is very small, but when it is added together with some of the other eight billion cells it produces enough of a wave to be recognized by an electroencephalographer, a doctor who reads these tracings. They tell whether a person has epilepsy, brain tumors, certain types of strokes, concussions, and many other conditions of the brain. This is a painless test except for the pain experienced when the eighteen to twenty-five needles are inserted into the scalp, just into the subcutaneous tissue. The patient does not need to be put to sleep for the test, but frequently it is desirable because this is the only way you can pick up certain brain tumors and some forms of epilepsy. At times the doctor will even give the patient a sleeping pill to put him to sleep.

This test is very similar to an electrocardiogram in that it is a test to pick up the electrical activity of an organ, in this case, the brain. Brain wave tests take sometimes one-half to two hours, depending on how much of a tracing the doctor desires and whether the patient is going to be put to sleep.

One does not have to be put into the hospital to have this test. It can be performed in a physician's office. Do not think your physician thinks you are a neurotic or an epileptic just because he orders this test. He may be looking for other diseases. He may want to exclude the possibility that you have a convulsive disorder. He also does not necessarily think you have a brain tumor just because he orders this test.

Cholesterol

Today, many patients are being sent to the laboratory by their family doctors for a blood test for cholesterol. If the level of the cholesterol is high in their blood they are placed on a low-cholesterol or low-fat diet. Recently a new drug has been developed to reduce it. Therefore patients have many questions about what cholesterol is and what to do about it.

What is cholesterol?

Cholesterol is a fat. There are three important blood fats: cholesterol, phospholipids and triglycerides. Also there is a small amount of free fatty acids in the blood. Cholesterol is found mostly in animal foods, such as meat, milk, and eggs. It is very important in forming the walls of our cells. Cholesterol is also used by the body to form certain hormones and bile acids, which are important for digestion of foods. There are other important things that cholesterol does in the body that I will not go into. The normal range of the blood cholesterol varies from one laboratory to another. It usually runs from between one hundred fifty to two hundred fifty milligrams per one hundred cubic centimeters of blood. Today most doctors order an analysis of all important blood fats: cholesterol, triglyceride, and phospholipid. In addition you may have blood drawn for lipoprotein, which is the protein that binds these blood fats so that they will not be easily absorbed by the tissues except under circumstances that the body desires. A high cholesterol usually is between four hundred and six hundred milligrams, but moderate elevations in cholesterol are found in many Americans, between two hundred fifty and four hundred milligrams. It is often difficult to make clear to patients that a thirty- to forty-point elevation is not too serious.

What causes a high blood cholesterol and what can I do about it?

There are five basic things that contribute to a high blood cholesterol. The first and probably the most important is heredity. This, of course, we cannot do much about. The other four factors that elevate the blood cholesterol we can do something about. First of all there is smoking. Smoking elevates the blood cholesterol about thirty to forty points and in some people even a little more. This is, of course, heavy smoking (one pack or more a day).

Second of all, a diet rich in cholesterol will elevate the blood cholesterol in people that have a hereditary predisposition for this. The quantity of food is as important as the quality. Therefore in a high-calorie diet the body converts both sugar and protein into cholesterol. Once cholesterol gets into or is formed in the body it cannot be excreted, except for a half gram to one gram a day through the intestinal tract. Some of it, as mentioned above, is converted into hormones and bile acids. Therefore, remember that when you take cholesterol in, it is not going to get out and it has to accumulate somewhere in your body. The dangerous thing is accumulation on the arteries, causing strokes and heart attacks. One must not only concentrate on reducing the amount of cholesterol in his diet. He must also keep from overeating, so that the sugar and protein taken in are not converted into cholesterol. In this sense a two thousand-calorie steak, which most people feel is low in cholesterol, would be just as dangerous as eating a big hunk of fat if ingested at one meal. Even someone who is an alcoholic and eats very little may develop a high cholesterol if he ingests four to five thousand calories of alcohol a day; this is not hard to do when one considers that a fifth of Scotch contains about three thousand calories.

A third important controllable factor causing an increase in cholesterol is lack of exercise. Walking one mile may burn only a slice of bread in an efficient human being, but this is still a slice of bread that could go into forming blood cholesterol. Regular exercise daily will also reduce body tension and stimulate the heart to circulate the blood cholesterol to areas where it is needed. The final controllable factor causing a high cholesterol is nervous tension. Some people, of course, smoke to relieve nervous tension but they are fooling themselves, because the nicotine may make them even more excited and nervous.

Electrocardiogram

What is an electrocardiogram?

An electrocardiogram is a recording of the electrical activity of your heart made by attaching electrodes from an electrocardiograph machine to your body. Just before each of your heartbeats, your heart gives off a wave of electrical activity. Your heart is like a large electrical cell, and just before each of the heartbeats this "cell" is discharged and gives off an electrical wave. It is very easy for an electrocardiograph to pick this up because your heart is so big. You could not, of course, get an electrical shock by putting your hand in front of your heart. Normally your heart beats between sixty to one hundred beats per minute, and therefore on the electrocardiograph recording there are sixty to one hundred electrical discharges per minute. An electrocardiogram can tell us whether the heart is beating too fast or too slow, which you could also pick up by a pulse beat. More important, when the heart is beating irregularly or extremely fast, the electrocardiogram will show why. The electrocardiogram can also tell us whether the heart is enlarged and also whether there is actual damage in certain areas of the heart, as occurs in heart attacks. The electrocardiogram cannot always tell us whether the coronary arteries are in spasm or partially blocked, but it usually tells us when the coronary arteries are completely blocked by a blood clot.

A person who has just had a normal electrocardiogram could have a heart attack the same evening or the same day. The person might then say that the physician had missed the diagnosis because he did not know how to read the electrocardiogram. This is not true. The only certain way to know whether a person has a predisposition to having a heart attack within the near future is to do a coronary angiogram, which involves injecting dye into the arteries of the heart to show whether there is a blockage. But your doctor may ask you to perform an *exercise electrocardiogram* (Master's two-step, as it is called professionally), a test where he takes an electrocardiogram immediately after you have exercised. This may show that you have a partial blockage of the coronary arteries or a "spasm" of the coronary arteries, but not always. On routine health examinations, particularly in executives, we do this test because we want to know whether they are going to have a heart attack in the very near future. Each individual patient naturally would want to know this. If you are concerned about whether you may be predisposed to having a heart attack, ask your doctor to perform an exercise electrocardiogram on you.

Many other diseases of the heart may be determined by doing an electrocardiogram. In addition, the doctor uses the electrocardiogram to determine whether you have too much or too little digitalis, an important heart pill that he prescribes for congestion of the heart and chest. The electrocardiogram is a painless test; it does not require hospitalization; and it does not require a person to be put under an anesthetic. We recommend electrocardiograms yearly on everyone over forty. Anyone who has had any type of heart disease should have an electrocardiogram every six months.

"Pap" Smear

What is a "Pap" smear?

A "Pap" smear is a technique devised by Papanicolaou, for whom it is named, to make slides from cervical, vaginal and uterine secretions to determine the presence of cancer of the womb.

Who should have this test?

All women from sixteen to one hundred should have this test performed once a year. In women with a strong family history of cancer it should be performed more often. Actually very few women have this test before they are married, and most older women avoid having it. This is foolish but understandable, in view of the slowly dying puritanical customs of our society. Men do not need this test. (Try and get it!?!)

How is it performed?

After you are undressed and properly draped and set in the stirrups on the examining table, a vaginal speculum is lubricated and gently inserted into the vagina (lower portion of the birth canal). Then, with a smooth applicator stick specially shaped for this purpose, the doctor scrapes the secretions around the cervix (mouth of the womb) and vagina and applies them to a glass slide. These slides are sprayed with a fixing solution and sent to the pathologist, who will examine them the next day and send a report to your doctor. Your doctor will then call you or mail you a report. After the slides are made, the vaginal speculum is removed and your doctor will often examine your womb and other female organs with his finger. He will also do a breast examination, to look for tumors.

What if I don't have a "Pap" test yearly?

Most likely nothing will happen to you. However, one in every two hundred women examined has cancer and you may be that one.

Physical Examination

Why should I have a physical examination?

It has been shown by statistical analysis of a large number of physical examinations performed on healthy people over the years that at least in thirty to forty percent of these physicals some unknown disease has been detected. The most important part of medical care is not treating disease but in helping people who are healthy stay healthy. Therefore I recommend periodic physical examinations for all children from one to a hundred years old. Just how often a physical examination should be performed on people who assume themselves to be healthy is a matter of opinion. It is my opinion it should be performed at least every two years and preferably every year.

What should the physical examination consist of?

A good physical examination should consist of a complete medical history on the patient and complete examination of the eyes, ear, nose and throat, neck, chest, heart, abdomen, a rectal on everyone, and a vaginal on females. The extremities are checked for the character of the pulses, varicose veins, and bone or joint abnormalities. It should also include a neurological examination.

Let me describe how physical examinations are handled in my office. You will come to the office with a urine specimen preferably a freshly voided morning specimen, and this will be taken by the nurse as she greets you. She will then have the laboratory technician draw blood for sugar, cholesterol, complete blood count, and for a few other tests. If you desire an executive-type examination, a cardiogram, chest x-ray, and pulmonary function test are also performed. (See table of contents for reference to specific tests.)

Then you are taken to an examining room, where the nurse takes your blood pressure and records your weight and height. Then she asks you several questions about your past history. She will want to know if you have ever had diabetes, tuberculosis, asthma, blood disease, kidney or liver diseases, etc. She will want to know the diseases of your father, mother, brothers and sisters, etc. She will ask you about any complaints you might have in each of your organs, beginning with your eyes, ears, nose, and working down to your heart and stomach. She will ask you about any defects that you know you have and about previous operations, accidents or hospitalizations.

After this you are taken to my office, where you will sit down and go over this history with me more thoroughly. More important I will ask you if you have any specific complaints that are bothering you at the present time. If you do then each one of these complaints, whether it be a headache, chest pain or fatigue, will be investigated in depth by further questions. Some of these questions may seem a bit ridiculous but you should answer them and realize this is only to help you.

After I have reviewed your history with you, the nurse will put you back in an examination room again, and you will take off all of your clothes except for your underwear or shorts. You will take off your shoes and socks, as well, because every doctor wants to see your feet. Sometimes he will spot athlete's foot or flat feet or some unusual clubbing of your toenails, which will help him diagnose an important disease. While you are freezing in the examining room I will come in and examine you. Usually we try to put a sheet around the patient so that he won't freeze.

The first thing I do is look at the eyes with an ophthalmoscope. This is a little instrument that has a special set of lenses and a special light that can shine right through your pupil and reflect the back of your eyes to the doctor. He can then see the blood vessels at the back of your eyes and also your optic nerve, which is the only nerve in your body that he can see directly. The most important purpose of the ophthalmoscopic examination is to show the character of the blood vessels; we can tell how much fat you have on your arteries, whether there are hemorrhages from your arteries or veins, and whether there are any unusual abnormalities of these arteries or veins. This tells a lot about the rest of your body. By looking at the optic nerve we can tell whether there is increased pressure in the brain (a sign of a brain tumor). By flicking the lenses on the ophthalmoscope we can tell roughly whether you need glasses or not. I then shoot a light into your pupils to see whether they react properly. There are ten or fifteen different diseases that may be diagnosed by finding an abnormality of the pupils. By looking at the conjunctiva I can tell whether you are anemic.

Then I look at the ears, the drums especially, with an otoscope. I can tell whether you have had a lot of infection of your drums in your childhood. I can see any recent or present inflammation in your drums. In some patients I discover that they have a perforated drum that they never knew about. With a tuning fork I can tell whether the hearing is equal in both ears, and if there is some inequality I know that the patient needs an audiogram, which will give more definite information about his hearing.

Examination of the mouth including the tongue and the throat is performed to see if the tonsils are normal or if the tongue shows any atrophy, which might indicate anemia or other diseases. (The tongue used to be a very important indicator for the old country doctor.)

After examining the tongue and the throat, the neck is examined, and here I look for enlargement of the lymph glands, which are important in finding disease. They are frequently enlarged if there is inflammation in the nose, throat, tonsils, etc. They are also enlarged in infectious mononucleosis. Also in the neck I feel the thryoid to see if it is enlarged and to check for tumors on the thyroid. By looking at the neck I can see whether the veins are distended, as this may be an indication that there is heart failure.

Proceeding on I will pick up my stethoscope and place it over the chest and examine it front to back to listen for any unusual noises in the chest and also to see if the patient has normal breathing. By tapping the chest wall I can tell whether there is any fluid or any unusual masses in the lung itself, even though I can't feel them. If I have the patient say certain words, like "ninety-nine," I can feel vibrations through the chest wall that tell me whether there is fluid or a collapse of the lung, etc. Next, using the stethoscope and the hand I examine the heart. The hand is placed over the left side of the chest to feel for the point of maximum pulsation of the heart, which tells me how large the heart is. I tap the area of the chest over the heart to find if the heart is enlarged. Then by listening with the stethoscope I can hear murmurs and any unusual changes in the heart sounds, which would indicate rheumatic fever, a heart attack, or some congenital anomaly of the heart. The breasts are examined.

Then I proceed to lay the patient flat on the table on his back and feel the abdomen. The most important part of examining the abdomen is *palpation.* I put my fingers under the left ribs to feel for the spleen and under the right ribs to feel for the liver. Usually these are not palpated unless enlarged. I then feel the sides of the abdomen and the loins for the kidneys. After this the entire abdomen is palpated to look for any abnormal masses or tumors or any tenderness that might indicate a peptic ulcer or appendicitis, etc.

Then I have the patient stand so that I can feel for hernias, not just in the groin or testicles but also in the umbilicus (the navel). In the male the testicles are palpated to see if they are enlarged and the penis is examined to see if there are any unusual abnormalities or discharge. Then before doing a rectal and pelvic examination, the legs are examined, particularly for any edema (swelling). An indentation can be made with the finger on the lower part of the leg when there is real swelling from fluid. The joints are palpated for any cracking and the bones are examined. Then the pulses in the legs are examined around the feet. I look for varicose veins, flat feet, and other abnormalities in the shape of the legs or feet. From this I usually proceed to the neurological examination, which with the routine physical usually includes percussion of the reflexes with a percussion hammer, and this includes the biceps reflexes in the arms, the knee jerks and ankle jerks. The bottoms of the feet are stroked with a pointed instrument such as a pen to elicit a very important reflex called a Babinski sign. This is a certain indication of disease of the nervous system. With a tuning fork I can tell whether the vibratory sensation is intact in the arms and the legs. If this is absent it may be a sign of an unusual blood condition or more common neurological diseases, such as multiple sclerosis, or even a spinal cord tumor. I usually examine the touch and pain sensation with a pin or cotton.

After this the patient is again laid on the examining table, and if it is a female her feet are put into the stirrups and she is draped properly for a pelvic examination. I pass a speculum into the vagina, or the entrance to the womb (the speculum is sometimes a little cold but otherwise is not painful at all) and examine the mouth of the womb, which is an important place for cancer to develop. The mouth of the womb is scraped with a stick and the scrapings are put on a slide and sent away for pathological examination to catch early cancer. Sometimes washings of the vagina are taken with a bulb syringe, and this is placed on a slide and sent away for examination for the same reason. Then the speculum is withdrawn and I do a pelvic examination by the gloved hand. This is to determine the size of the womb and the ovaries and look for cancer and other diseases in that area. Then a rectal examination is performed with one finger to look for cancer, hemorrhoids, and in the male to feel the size of the prostate.

With an executive physical, after the rectum is adequately cleaned out a sigmoidoscopic examination is performed at the same time of the routine physical. The sigmoidoscopic examination will be described more fully in another chapter but generally this is done with a tube with a light on it that we pass up into the rectum to look for tumors and other diseases of the rectum and the sigmoid part of the large intestine.

This completes the physical examination, and if the patient can still walk after all this he can presume himself healthy without even hearing the doctor's report. However,

I like to give the patient the complete report of his lab work, x-rays, and physical examination at a follow-up visit to the office if he can be persuaded to return. Each patient is then provided with a written report of his examination so that he can take this with him wherever he goes.

The doctor may find abnormalities on the examination that require further diagnostic tests, such as x-rays and lab work, and of course the patient is asked to come back for these. Sometimes the patient has a family doctor following his progress who must get a report of each routine periodical physical. In this day and age the patient should know everything the doctor finds on the examination, because after all he is the one that has to live with it. However, it is unnecessary to tell a patient that he has cancer, even if one is certain about it, unless you are asked. I usually use a less fearful term such as "tumor," because invariably the patient can accept this more readily.

Some executive physicals include an x-ray of the stomach, which is performed by swallowing a white chalk barium substance and taking several x-rays, and a gall bladder series (an x-ray of the gall bladder). They may include an x-ray of the kidneys, in which we inject a dye into the veins in the arm and after five to ten minutes take films from over the abdomen to observe the dye going through the kidneys. It is unnecessary to have these special examinations every year. Some people even question that a chest x-ray is necessary every year, since cancer of the lungs develops so quickly that you could have a chest x-ray every three months and not catch it in time. I still feel that since there are so many other conditions in the chest that can be picked up by routine x-ray, it is very valuable on a yearly basis.

Premarital Examination

To most patients a premarital examination is simply a "blood test." It is appalling how many patients expect their doctor to simply fill out a form certifying that they are clean from venereal disease with just the "blood test" from the local laboratory without a complete physical examination. I frequently have patients call me up and ask if I will simply sign the form without a physical. This I refuse to do. Both parties in the marriage should have a complete physical examination to rule out venereal disease, including gonorrhea and syphilis. A blood test will not exclude the possibility of gonorrhea, lymphogranuloma inguinale, or lymphogranuloma venereum. In addition a physical examination on the female and male will help determine whether each of them can have children. It might be even wise for the male to have a sperm count. In this way we can determine before marriage whether the male is fit to have children. I think both persons should be advised of any physical defects in the other prior to marriage. For instance if one of the two has diabetes this should be determined before the marriage and not after it. Thus a thorough physical examination should be done on both parties.

Beyond this I think any premarital examination should include a thorough discussion with each person separately and then with the two together on the differences between a man and woman, both sexually and otherwise. As I have pointed out in my discussion on marriage, the female is usually less active sexually. She requires intercourse perhaps two or three times a month while the male would like to have it two to three times a day. This is not because the male is oversexed or she is undersexed. It is just simply a physiological difference between the two. In addition certain methods have to be used to build a female up to a climax, whereas the male takes very little time to reach a climax. The differences between how the female and male react in a climax should be explained. I like to give couples a book on sexual techniques so that they both understand how to keep each other happy sexually. An excellent book for these purposes is *Ideal Marriage,* by Dr. Theodor H. Van De Velde (New York: Random House, 1965).

The emotional differences between the sexes should be explained. The fact that the woman is depressed at the time of her period must be noted so that the male can understand why she sometimes gets very hostile toward him for no apparent reason. I try to tell the woman how to keep the man happy by showing him a lot of respect, by treating him nicely during illness, by making him feel that he is the boss (even if she doesn't feel he is). Beyond this the two should be examined regarding their compatibility. Any religious, intellectual, social, or financial incompatibilities should be discussed, because only before marriage can these be worked out adequately. If it is found that there is marked incompatibility, even if they are madly in love with each other, they should be referred for counseling. Sometimes the physician himself can do it, but if not a marriage counselor should be contacted. A physician should state whether he recommends marriage or not.

Finally, although most couples are too shy to ask about birth control at this time, this should be thoroughly discussed so that the woman can be fitted for a diaphragm or given contraceptive cream or birth control pills prior to the time of their honeymoon and thus prevent one of the worst crises in marriages: having a baby too soon.

Such an examination as I have here described would take at least an hour. Most physicians find this too much time to spend away from stamping out disease. However, when one considers that there have been over nine million divorces since the second world war, one realizes that a little bit of preventive medicine in this area would certainly be of tremendous value in our society. It is far too easy to get married in our society. In addition to the premarital examination suggested here, engaged couples should be required to attend a series of lectures on marriage. A waiting period of at least six months should be mandatory between the time a couple get a marriage license and the time they can get married. If a learner's permit is necessary prior to receiving a driver's license, why shouldn't a similar procedure be required in marriage, a potentially more dangerous "vehicle"?

Sigmoidoscopy

What is a sigmoidoscopy?

A sigmoidoscopy is an examination with a sigmoidoscope, which is a hollow metal tube with a light on the end of it used for looking into the rectum and the lower portion of the large bowel (the sigmoid part of the colon).

Why do I have to have a sigmoidoscopy?

Usually your doctor wants to do a sigmoidoscopy because he suspects you may have a tumor of the rectum or the colon, or that you may have some inflammatory condition of the rectum or large bowel, such as inflamed hemorrhoids or colitis. However, sigmoidoscopy is being performed frequently on a routine basis to catch cancer early before it may cause symptoms. This is particularly valuable in people over forty years of age, when the incidence of polyps and tumors of the rectum and colon increases remarkably. Therefore, if you go for a periodic health physical you will probably have a sigmoidoscopy.

What is the procedure of examining a patient with a sigmoidoscope?

Usually the doctor will have you take an enema an hour or two before the examination. Then you will lay down on the examining table with your rear end propped up in the air, or you may be put on a specially built table, such as the Ritter table, which will help the doctor prop your rear end up in the air with your rectum exposed. Then he will put greasy material on his glove and insert his index finger into your rectum to make sure your rectum is clean and to be sure there is nothing that might obstruct the passing of the scope. Next he will lubricate the scope, which is not much bigger than your index finger, with greasy material, and he will pass the scope into the rectum gently for about two to three inches. Then he will remove the obturator from the instrument (a rounded plug which facilitated putting the instrument into your rectum for the first two to three inches) and will insert the instrument further under direct vision, making sure that it passes only in the lumen (the inside of the rectum and colon).

He may have to pump air into your rectum to flatten out the folds of your rectum that may impede the passage of the instrument. After he has passed the instrument approximately twelve to fifteen inches, he will withdraw the instrument slowly and take a second look at everything that he saw on the way in. In this way he will often see tumors that he missed before. Then the scope is withdrawn and the examination is completed. You will probably pass air after the examination and sometimes during the examination, but do not be embarrassed because this is common and both the doctor and his assistant are used to it. They are not embarrassed at all.

Is a sigmoidoscopy dangerous?

No. It is not any more dangerous than using an instrument to look into any other area of your body, such as the vagina or the ear, if it is performed by a competent operator.

Urine Test

Doctors of twenty to thirty years ago almost invariably asked patients to bring a urine sample with them whenever they had an office call. At that time the urine was tested only for sugar (to catch diabetes) and for albumin (to pick up kidney disease and high blood pressure). Yet today the urine is less frequently examined, when, paradoxically, more can be found on a urine sample than ever before. Why don't doctors ask for the urine more frequently today? Probably the main reason is that we have sophisticated blood tests, but this makes the urine test no less important. Today we can pick up sugar in the urine by a simple test. We can pick up albumin, which would indicate kidney disease, heart disease or hypertension; we can pick up red cells, which might indicate a bleeding disorder or kidney disease, and white cells, which may indicate infection of the kidney or bladder. By testing the weight of the urine in comparison to water (called specific gravity), we are able to find out how well the kidneys can function or whether they are diseased. But beyond these tests we can use a urine sample to determine how much hormone a patient has in his blood, not just hormones from the adrenal glands but also hormones from the reproductive organs and the pituitary, etc. Furthermore, we can test the urine for excessive excretion of copper, lead, and other heavy metals, and we are able to find out whether a person is on certain drugs, which is important today. So the urine sample is extremely important. The doctor may ask for a twenty-four hour sample when testing for some of the above more sophisticated substances. It is also important to have a twenty-four-hour urine to tell how much urine you are putting out. Many patients notice when they void they have blood in their urine, and, of course, this can indicate disease of the prostate, bladder or kidney. It is frequently due to menstruation in females. Other patients notice a very dark urine. Often this has nothing to do with disease in the urinary tract. A dark urine can indicate that the patient is developing jaundice or it can indicate that there is bleeding high up in the urinary tract. It may indicate that the patient has some hereditary disease. There is no cause to panic when one passes dark urine. The patient is wise to get a urine test by his physician.

A cloudy urine is usually normal, because if one eats a lot of phosphates in his diet or a lot of calcium he may excrete cloudy urine. A cloudy urine may also indicate pus cells in the urine. These can be seen when examined by the physician under the microscope. Cloudy urine may indicate that there is an excess secretion of calcium and uric acid. Uric acid is important in the diagnosis of gout. Unusual colors of the urine such as green, orange, and chartreuse may be found but these are usually insignificant. Some of the drugs that are prescribed for urinary tract disease may color the urine blue or orange, and if your physician has not warned you of this before it may alarm you unnecessarily. It is important to emphasize in closing that any unusual change in your urine should not cause alarm until you have discussed it with your physician.

X-ray Examinations

What are x-ray examinations?

X-rays are one of the most important diagnostic examinations available to doctors today. An x-ray is like a light ray except that it can penetrate through the skin and even to some extent through the bones of the body; therefore, with them the doctor can see structures underneath the skin. Before the use of films the doctor applied the x-rays to a fluoroscopic screen so that he could look at your internal organs through the screen, but now with films he can make a permanent impression. X-rays are not dangerous, and a person can have up to thirty chest x-rays a year without getting a dose of x-ray likely to produce cancer. As you know x-rays are actually used in the treatment of cancer. Many people have large doses of x-ray for the treatment of cancer but rarely develop additional cancer in another part of their body as a result of the x-rays. Radiologists are exposed to x-rays for years and the vast majority of them never develop any serious cancer. So, do not be alarmed by the number of pictures your doctor may take. The very fast film that is used today allows us to take more x-rays with less exposure to get the same result.

The chest x-ray

The chest x-ray is becoming part of every periodic examination. It is also being made available to the public through mobile units at no charge. This is because the x-ray of the chest is so vital in picking up tuberculosis of the lungs, enlargement of the heart, and cancer of the lungs. The technician will place the patient in front of a fourteen-by-seven-teen-inch film and then turn the x-ray machine beam on and pass it through the chest to expose the film. Then the film is developed and a pretty good reproduction of the organs of the chest is produced. Hundreds of diseases can be picked up in this way, chest disease as well as heart disease. This is a painless procedure and does not require any special preparation. It takes about two to three minutes to perform.

Gastrointestinal series

This is an x-ray of the esophagus, the stomach, and the small intestine. With delayed films a picture of the large intestines can also be taken. It is more commonly called an x-ray of the stomach, but as you can see it includes a lot more than that. With this the doctor can discover cancers, ulcers, and inflammations of the esophagus, stomach, duodenum, and small intestines. The most common reason for employing this procedure is to see if you have an ulcer.

The procedure for this examination is as follows: First, you eat no food from midnight before the examination; that means no breakfast on the morning of the examination. Then you go to the hospital or doctor's office and undress and put on a gown. In the x-ray room you swallow a glass of white liquid called barium sulfate; while this is going through the esophagus and stomach the doctor will take spot pictures of the passage of this material. He will press your stomach and try to get the material to pass into all of the areas of the stomach and intestines and esophagus to make sure there is no ulcer or tumor in these areas. He will put you in different positions on the fluoroscopic table and snap anywhere from ten to twenty films during this procedure. The procedure usually takes about fifteen minutes to one-half hour for the initial fluoroscoping and shooting the films and then you often must come back in two hours for a delayed film. In between the initial portion of the examination and the late film you can go about your business and relax, but you must not eat or drink anything. After the procedure is over you can eat. It is wise to take a laxative to get the barium out of your system. The only possible harm in this examination is that the barium could get jammed in the large intestine and cause a partial intestinal obstruction, but this is unusual. There is no great harm from the x-rays themselves. It is unusual for people to be allergic to the barium.

Barium enema

This is an x-ray examination of the large bowel and rectum. The doctor can also see the terminal portion of the small intestine on many occasions. This allows the doctor to see cancer, inflammation and ulcers of the large intestine more clearly than he would on the G. I. (gastrointestinal) series.

The procedure in this case is to refrain from eating after midnight on the night before and also to take castor oil to clean out the intestinal tract. If you are not clean after the castor oil, then it may be necessary to have a cleansing enema, either with saline or soap suds. The following morning you report to the physician's office or hospital and undress and put on a gown. A tube is put up into the rectum and barium sulfate is pumped into the rectum to fill the entire large intestine. The doctor looks at your abdomen in a dark room with a fluoroscope and takes spot films while the barium is being pushed in and as it comes out. He may press your stomach and your lower abdomen to push the barium into areas that are difficult to fill spontaneously. After he has taken his pictures then you may go to the bathroom and evacuate the barium sulfate. This is a very innocuous procedure and the only serious danger is if the barium becomes hardened and obstructs the intestine, which is rare. An enema will usually relieve any obstruction of this nature. There is no need to be put into the hospital for this procedure. You can go about your business once the pictures are taken.

X-ray of the gall bladder

This is often referred to as a gall-bladder series or *cholecystogram.* In this procedure dye tablets taken by mouth are absorbed by and concentrated in the gall bladder. Pictures of this can be taken to show gall stones, inflammation of the gall bladder, and occasionally tumors of the gall bladder, which are rare. The most important reason for doing this procedure is to look for gall stones. The procedure in this examination is to eat nothing after supper the night before. Then take between ten and fourteen tablets of the dye by mouth, swallowing them with water the night before. Withhold your breakfast the morning of the examination and go to the physician's office or hospital. Here, after undressing and putting on a gown, you are taken into the x-ray room and films are taken of the gall bladder in different positions. The x-ray beam and films will be placed adjacent to the abdomen. After the initial films you are requested to drink a "milk shake"-like substance, and another series of films is taken to see if the gall bladder has contracted and emptied properly upon the stimulus of a fatty meal (the "milk shake"). This is a very painless procedure. There is no serious danger from the pills, although you may get diarrhea and occasionally an allergic reaction with hives. The procedure does not have to be performed in the hospital. You may go about your business shortly after and do as you please. The time for this examination is approximately fifteen minutes for the initial films and then after drinking the "milk shake" another five to ten minutes to take further films. You can be in and out of the physician's office or hospital within one hour. The doctor does not need to be present during this examination. It can all be performed entirely by the radiological technician.

The kidney x-ray

This is commonly called the *intravenous pyelogram* in professional circles. This is to determine if there are cancers, stones, or inflammation of the kidneys, bladder, and the ureters, and also enlargements or tumors of the prostate. The most important reason for giving this examination is to look for evidence of stones or tumors in the kidneys or bladder.

The procedure for this test is as follows: First the patient takes castor oil the night before the examination and withholds all food after midnight. He then reports to the physician's office or the hospital the following morning without breakfast. After the patient has undressed and put on a gown a preliminary scout film of the abdomen is taken. Then 20 to 30 cc. of dye is injected into the vein of one or the other arm, after first giving a test dose of 1 cc. of the dye or after giving a drop of the dye in the eye or an intradermal (skin) injection of the dye. Then shortly after the dye is injected films are taken of the kidney to see just how quickly the dye gets to each kidney and also to see the configuration of the kidneys, ureters, and bladder. Films are usually taken at five, ten and twenty minutes, and possibly at one hour. The patient may take most of this lying down but one of the pictures, at least, will be taken standing up to see how well the kidneys are evacuated by gravity. There are departures from the standard procedure in cases of people with high blood pressure, when films at one, three, and five minutes are taken, and in cases of other special problems that are too numerous to mention.

There is possibly a little more danger in this examination than in the others I have mentioned, not because of the x-ray exposure but because of the injection of the dye intravenously. The patient may be allergic to the dye and go into shock. He should always be questioned as to whether he is allergic to iodine, seafoods, or other substances. The type of shock experienced is an anaphylactoid shock, which could cause him to become unconscious and possibly die (one in fifty thousand cases). The usual allergic reaction is just hives or a rash and can easily be cured by a shot of epinephrine or cortisone. In most physicians' offices and hospitals where this procedure is performed, there is emergency equipment available to take care of this type of reaction. In any case the incidence of this reaction is less than an allergic reaction to penicillin, and people certainly do not hesitate to ask their doctors to give them penicillin. This procedure does not need to be performed in the hospital if the doctor's office is equipped properly to handle the allergic reactions. After the examination you can go about your business and get something to eat. The dye does not remain in the system more than a day, except under unusual circumstances. The time for the performance of this examination is approximately one hour.

X-rays of the bones

X-rays of the bones are probably the most valuable diagnostic procedure in x-ray. In fact, they were the first reason that the x-ray was used. X-rays of the skull, spine, and bones of the extremities are taken by the hundreds every day in most hospitals. These are completely innocuous and only take one to two minutes to perform. The most common reason for taking x-rays of the bones is to look for fractures, but cancer of the bone can also be diagnosed, as well as certain metabolic diseases of the bone. Because of medicolegal implications, however, x-rays of the bones are being taken more frequently to be sure that one does not miss a hairline fracture of the skull or some other part of the body that might bring a lawsuit against the physician. It is foolish for a patient to be exposed to unnecesssary x-rays, but the legal profession has imposed this on us to a large extent. I personally think that if patients were not so quick to sue the doctor we would have a lot fewer x-rays of the bones and joints being performed.

The procedure is simple. The part of the body is exposed and any metal object must be removed, such as a wrist watch or glasses. The x-ray beam is directed on it and the film placed adjacent to that part of the body being x-rayed. As I said above, the time for this procedure is two or three minutes or less. Special views, however, are sometimes needed, so the patient may be required to come back for more films if the initial films do not show what the doctor is looking for.

Other x-rays

Today we can x-ray many other parts of the body, but since these are not routine I have not included them in this discussion. However, the reader should note that the same type of dye that is used for an intravenous pyelogram (Hypaque) and its derivatives can be used to light up the arteries in any part of the body, to light up the heart and its various chambers, and to light up the veins in any part of the body. With this material, therefore, we can find clots in the veins or arteries, whether it be the coronary or the cerebral arteries; and we can also see disturbances in the configuration of the arteries by tumors in many parts of the body, including the brain and the kidney, etc. These procedures, however, carry with them a greater risk of allergic reaction to the dye because larger amounts of dye are used. They also carry with them the risk of placing a needle in an artery. The needle may cause dislodgement of a piece of fat or calcium from the artery or cause a clot to form at the site of entry. It can also cause rupture of the artery. Depending on the skill of the person putting the needle into the artery or vein, these complications are pretty unusual. These procedures are sometimes performed under general anesthesia, and this carries with it the risks of anesthesia, which I will discuss in other sections.

Radioisotopes

Another important x-ray examination is a scan with the use of radioisotopes. A radioisotope is the form of an element that emits radiation. This is not always x-ray radiation. Gamma rays are the most important radiation for use in the diagnosis of disease. By attaching the element to a substance that can be selectively absorbed by the tissue to be examined, such as the thyroid, the element will concentrate in that tissue. A special type of Geiger counter placed over that tissue can outline its borders. This is a harmless procedure in that only very small amounts of the radioactive substance need be ingested or injected into the body. Once that is done the patient has only to lie still while the "Geiger counter" passes over the organ to be examined and counts the amount of radiation coming from that organ. In this way the thyroid may be examined by ingesting radioactive iodine; the brain may be examined by injecting either mercury or technetium into the veins; and the liver may be examined by injecting gold or rose bengal, etc. The entire procedure takes one to two hours. It is usually unnecessary to fast before this procedure. However, if the patient cannot lie still this procedure is inaccurate. This procedure is most valuable in diagnosing tumors, such as tumors of the thyroid, brain, or liver. It can also help diagnose other conditions in these organs. Radioisotopes are also used to treat tumors as well. For example, they are used to treat chronic leukemias and tumors of the thyroid.

MEDICATIONS AND TREATMENTS

Anesthesia

Anesthesia may be local, spinal, or general. *Local anesthesia* (usually Novocain or one of its relatives) is injected around the area to be incised. Some patients can even undergo abdominal surgery under local. There are few complications from local anesthesia; these are allergy to Novocain and Novocain toxicity.

Spinal anesthesia

The drug used in this form of anesthesia is also Novocain and its derivatives. It is given through a special needle inserted at the base of the spine. The Novocain spreads up the spinal column to the level of anesthesia desired. One may safely anesthetize a person from the chest down. Abdominal surgery may be performed easily with this technique. Many obstetricians use it for deliveries. Contrary to popular belief, a spinal tap is not dangerous at all. I have done over ten thousand of them without a single serious complication.

General anesthesia

We have come a long way since chloroform was introduced as the first clinically useful general anesthetic. Its margin of safety was narrow. Ether is still used but it has been largely replaced by fluethane, which is associated with much less postoperative nausea and vomiting and other problems. Good anesthesia is also obtained with Sodium Pentothal, but since there is laryngospasm an endotracheal tube may be used if the procedure is to be long. Laughing gas (nitrous oxide) is still used for induction (first stage of anesthesia). The best induction is the warm voice of the anesthesiologist and the patient's confidence in the surgeon.

When you are to have a surgical procedure don't hesitate to ask your doctor what anesthetic he plans and mention your preference. He can't always suit you but he will try. Any drug allergies should be mentioned also.

Aspirin

What is aspirin?

Aspirin is technically acetylsalicylic acid, which comes in a white powder and is dispensed in the form of a tablet and occasionally can be dispensed in the form of a suppository to be administered by rectum. Aspirin is one of the most valuable drugs ever to be discovered and is useful in many illnesses.

What does it do?

Aspirin is both an analgesic, which means that it can combat pain, and a drug that will reduce fever. It also can combat inflammation, whatever it may be from. Finally, it also works as a very weak antibiotic.

What is aspirin used for?

I'm sure that the average reader has used aspirin many, many times in his life time. There were over fifty billion aspirins sold in the United States in the past year. Aspirin is useful in pain originating from any origin. Therefore it may be used in headaches, chest pain, joint pain, muscle pains, etc. However, if the pain is coming from the stomach or intestines the aspirin may irritate the situation and cause more pain than it will help. Aspirin is used frequently to bring fever down, especially in infants, who have such high fevers with even the most simple illnesses. Aspirin is used as a specific anti-inflammatory agent in a variety of diseases. These include rheumatic fever, rheumatoid arthritis, osteoarthritis, gout, the common cold and influenza.

Is it dangerous?

Aspirin in the proper dosage, five to ten grains or one to two tablets three or four times a day, is not usually dangerous. However, we find that some patients are very sensitive to aspirin. They may get gastritis, or inflammation of the stomach; they may get a thinning effect in their blood, causing bleeding or hemorrhaging; and occasionally they may get a pustular rash on the skin. Aspirin is also dangerous because infants frequently find the sugared pills tasty and ingest numerous pills, leading to acute intoxication. This is why if you are taking large amounts of aspirin you should be under the supervision of your physician. Many people in this country diagnose and medicate themselves, more than in any other country in the world, and aspirin is the drug that is most abused in this regard.

Blood Thinners

What are blood thinners?

Blood thinners are drugs that keep the blood from clotting too rapidly. They do not really thin the blood, as such, because they do not lower the number of red cells or white cells in the blood. Two drugs are commonly used for thinning the blood—heparin and Dicumarol. Heparin comes in a solution for injection, because if given by mouth it would be destroyed by the enzymes in the intestinal tract. Dicumarol comes in tablet form and can be given by mouth.

What do blood thinners do?

Blood thinners, as stated above, prevent the blood from clotting. Heparin does this by interfering with the action of the platelets, or small clotting cells in the blood, and also by interfering with the action of three or four different clotting factors in the blood. However, Dicumarol does this primarily by affecting one clotting factor—prothrombin.

What are blood thinners used for?

Blood thinners are used to thin the blood or decrease the "clotability" of the blood in patients who have a blood clot somewhere in their body. This includes heart attack victims, victims of strokes, and patients who have a clot in their legs, either in the veins or arteries.

Are blood thinners dangerous?

Blood thinners are potentially a very dangerous drug and cannot be used without the constant supervision of your physician. For years we did not allow heparin to be used outside of the hospital; but now, since we have more intelligent patients and better communication by phone with both the doctor and the hospital, even heparin can be used outside the hospital. We have been using Dicumarol outside the hospital for a number of years, and, as most patients know, we are able to regulate the amount of Dicumarol a patient takes by testing his blood once or twice a month. The test is called a prothrombin time. If a patient gets too much of either of these drugs he may hemorrhage from the mouth, from the stomach, or from any number of other organs in the body.

Catheters

The first time somebody said that they were going to catheterize me I had the shock of my life. I can imagine that all patients get the same feeling. Usually when we talk about catheterizing someone we refer to catheterizing the bladder by passing a tube through the penis or urethra, the canal that runs from the outside into the bladder in both male and female. In my mind this canal seems very small. I'm sure it seems very small in your mind, also. Believe it or not, the hole that one urinates through can be stretched enough to admit a gun barrel without much pain, although I wouldn't try it. The diameter of a catheter that a doctor or nurse inserts into your bladder is much smaller than this. In many cases it is much smaller than a soda straw. If it is done correctly there should be no pain at all experienced during this procedure.

The main reason that patients used to be catheterized was that they could not urinate. This was particularly important after an operation in which a patient was put to sleep and his bladder had gone to sleep, as well, and could not contract very effectively. Today because it is frequently important to get a sterile urine specimen, patients are catheterized just for a diagnosis. Many patients, particularly older men with prostate trouble in whom an operation has been unsuccessful or impossible to do, have to have a permanent catheter inserted. Also, paraplegics and victims of polio and other paralyzing conditions of the nervous system must have a permanent catheter. Those of you who have met such people know that they do not complain about the catheter being painful and do not shudder about having a new catheter placed in. Catheters are usually rubber or plastic and rarely cause any pain on insertion. A catheter can be attached to a bottle by means of some other tubing so that the urine can be collected continuously for twenty-four hours or an indefinite period of time. Following an operation on the prostate, or even the bladder, it is very important to keep a catheter in the bladder so that the urine will not distend the bladder and rupture the incision.

There are other types of catheters. There are rectal catheters, which we use to promote the release of gas from the intestinal tract, particularly after an operation; Levine tubes or catheters, which we place into the stomach to drain the acid out of the stomach or to introduce ice water or some other substance to help heal the stomach; and endotracheal tubes, a form of catheter that we introduce into the trachea or lungs so that we can control the respirations and put oxygen directly into the lungs. This is particularly useful during an operation when the respirations may be slowed or paralyzed altogether by the anesthetic. Today we put small catheters into the ear drum to keep the pressure from building up behind the drum and rupturing it, particularly in kids with ear infections. We put catheters into the veins to allow for continuous administration of intravenous fluid; in this way there is much less pain to the patient, because we do not have to insert needles every time we start a new intravenous fluid. Of course, if these catheters become blocked it is necessary to insert another catheter. We insert catheters into the arteries to inject dye and take x-rays of the arteries, so that we can demonstrate diseases of the arteries in various parts of the body. We may catheterize the carotid or a femoral artery, inject dye through these arteries and take pictures. A catheter may be passed all the way up the arteries or veins into the heart to inject the dye for subsequent x-rays of the heart to demonstrate the valves, etc. Following an operation on the gall bladder, a catheter may be placed in the common duct to allow for a good circulation of the bile and to allow any overflow of the bile to come out the catheter. In this way the bile will not back up into the liver or possibly rupture and go into the abdominal cavity.

Catheters or drains are often placed in infectious wounds in the abdomen or any other place in the body. This allows the surgeon to pump out the pus. When the patient has a rupture of his abdomen or chest wall, a catheter is often inserted to drain the blood or other fluids that accumulate, which would, of course, lead to infection if it were not removed. Also, in a rupture of the lung a catheter is placed in the chest to pump out the air that is constantly coming in. In spinal anesthesia the anesthesiologist may pass a catheter into the subarachnoid space, the area where the spinal fluid is located, and inject the anesthetic continuously to keep the lower half of the body numb. In babies who have watermelon heads (hydrocephalics) a catheter is passed from the area of the "water" accumulation in the brain into the jugular vein or other areas so that the "water" will drain off when the pressure gets too high. There are other uses for catheters in medicine that I will not go into at this time.

Circumcision

What is circumcision?

Circumcision is the removal of the foreskin of the penis, exposing the glans, or head of the penis. This is usually performed in the male, but in some countries, particularly in Africa, circumcision of the female is performed. In females the organ is called the clitoris.

For what reasons are circumcisions done?

Circumcisions used to be performed only to allow for urination and a complete and comfortable erection of the penis. However, it is well known today that the hygiene of the head of the penis is much better if the foreskin is removed to expose the head of the penis, so that a good cleaning of the entire organ can be accomplished. The Jewish people knew this thousands of years ago. It is well known that men who have had a circumcision have a lower incidence of cancer of the penis and also that in Jewish women, whose husbands are virtually all circumcised, there is a much lower incidence of cancer of the mouth of the womb. It is also likely that venereal disease is less frequent in men who are circumcised.

What is the operation like?

A circumcision can be done under local anesthesia, and in newborn infants no anesthesia may be used at all. However, most adults have the procedure performed under general anesthesia, because this is a sensitive organ. The doctor merely takes hold of the amount of foreskin that is to be removed and cuts it off, either using a circular clamp as a guide or under direct vision, and the edges of the remaining foreskin are sutured together. In other words, it is no more difficult than cutting a fold of skin from another part of the body.

Is it dangerous?

A circumcision is not dangerous and will in no way endanger your sex life or your ability to urinate if it is done by a competent surgeon.

Colostomy

What is a colostomy?

A colostomy is the incision of an opening for the large bowel on the anterior abdominal wall. You may also have an ileostomy, in which case the small intestine is allowed to open via the anterior abdominal wall.

Why do I have to have a colostomy?

The main reason for a colostomy is cancer of the large bowel. Usually the cancer is in the lower portion of the large bowel, and therefore an artificial rectum must be created on your anterior abdominal wall to bypass the area of the cancer in the lower bowel. (Most of the time the passage of the stool is obstructed by the cancer.) Other conditions of the large bowel may also require a colostomy, such as diverticulitis. In ulcerative colitis the entire large bowel may be resected and an ileostomy created. Sometimes severe infection of the rectum determines that the large bowel must be connected to the anterior abdominal wall temporarily until the infection is cleared, when it can be reconnected to the rectum.

How can I manage a colostomy?

The difficulty of a colostomy is that you have no means of preventing the passage of stools when you don't want it; therefore, you must wear a colostomy bag over the opening in the anterior abdominal wall at all times. Just like the rectum the colostomy can become obstructed by a hard piece of stool, and therefore you must be able to give yourself enemas at these times. With the newer colostomy bags and the new means of fitting them snugly to the abdominal wall, it is unusual to have any feces leak out around the bag, so that undesirable odors are infrequent. Many patients get extremely emotionally upset by a colostomy, but this is unnecessary if proper training is given to the patient. Many patients live a healthy and comfortable life with a colostomy bag. Your local cancer society can give you further instructions on the use of a colostomy.

Contraceptives

What is a contraceptive?

A contraceptive is a device or a medicine that is used to prevent conception. To be more concrete, it prevents the male sperm from fertilizing the female egg or prevents the development of sperm or egg in the male or female respectively. In this era of extreme population explosion, contraceptives have become more widely used, and I think they ought to be. It is foolish to bring more than four or five children per family into the world under the present conditions and the projection of population growth in the next century.

What types of contraceptives are there?

Well, there are eight types that are most commonly used: (1) a condom, or a rubber, which fits over the male penis; (2) the contraceptive creams, which are placed into the female vagina and immediately destroy the male sperm on contact so that they will not be able to reach the egg; (3) the diaphragm placed over the mouth of the womb; (4) an intrauterine device (IUD), which is inserted into the womb of the female and which in some way disturbs the ability of the fertilized egg to implant in the uterus, or else makes it difficult for the male sperm to reach the egg; (5) the douche, which can be used immediately following intercourse; (6) the rhythm method, by which a woman can take her temperature to determine when she will be laying an egg and therefore refrain from having intercourse during that period of time; (7) the method of "pulling out" (coitus interruptus), which is a method by which the male interrupts intercourse just at the time when he may eject the semen into the vagina; and (8), the most recent contraceptive device, "the pill," which the woman can take to prevent ovulation. We will discuss each of these devices and cite their advantages and disadvantages. (See also *Abortion,* page 304), and *Sterilization,* (page 318.)

THE CONDOM

This is a thin rubber sheath that fits over the penis. It measures between six and eight inches long. The best type has a receptacle at the end to collect the sperm. Those with a lubricant added are easiest to put on and allow for an easier insertion of the penis into the vagina. This method is almost a hundred percent effective if the condom fits snug. If the man has an incomplete erection it will not fit snug and may slip off, or the sperm may leak out. If he remains in the vagina after orgasm it may slip off on the way out. Condoms rarely burst. The disadvantages of a condom are that you must carry one with you, you must interrupt love-making to put it on, and neither the male nor female may get maximum sensitivity through the rubber barrier. Otherwise it is a good method of contraception, provided you observe the above precautions.

THE CONTRACEPTIVE CREAMS

There are various types of creams, suppositories and foam. One such cream is Delfen, which I usually recommend.

This cream is about ninety to ninety-five percent effective if used consistently. The difficulty in using the cream is that women must prepare themselves before undertaking any love-making by inserting the cream or foam into her vagina; or, if she desires to wait until she is certain that her lover is going to make an approach, she must interrupt the love-making and insert the cream. This is very embarrassing for some women, but the main difficulty is that some couples do not want to take the time to do this. The cream usually does not affect the male, but sometimes it will burn the end of the penis.

THE DIAPHRAGM

This is a large rubber plate inserted into the vagina and covering the mouth of the womb. Your doctor measures your cervical and vaginal diameter so it fits snug. It has the same disadvantages as the cream, and I do not recommend it.

THE INTRAUTERINE DEVICE

This plastic device can be inserted into your womb by your family physician for a charge of roughly twenty to thirty dollars right in his office. This device is ninety to ninety-five percent effective but some authorities claim ninety-seven percent effectiveness. There are various types, such as a coil, a bow, and also a ring and a button. In regard to intercourse these have no disadvantages at all. The device is always in place so that intercourse can be undertaken at any time of the day or night. The use of this device does not interrupt intercourse and it does not cause any pain to the male. The difficulties with the IUD are with the female; she may have excessive bleeding at the time of her normal menses, or she may have breakthrough bleeding occasionally. The device may also cause more cramps at the time of the menses and occasionally in between the periods. During the first couple of months of use the woman may not be safe, and she must constantly check the womb to make sure the device is still in place. Rarely the device may cause rupture of the womb and the device is displaced into the abdominal cavity. This is very unusual if the device is properly placed. I caution my patients about reading articles on the complications of such devices, as they are always extremely rare cases and a good deal of information is left out about the general health of the individual that has had the problem. In the woman who has never had a child the physician may have difficulty inserting an IUD, but generally women who have had two or more children do not have any difficulty with insertion. However, women who have had several children may have a tear of the mouth of the womb, and this may cause the device to be extruded more easily.

DOUCHING

Douching should be discouraged. It is of no benefit, because many times the sperm are ejected right into the mouth of the womb during intercourse. Women who use the douche method usually continue to have children.

RHYTHM

With the rhythm method the woman has to keep a temperature chart for about three to four months before she can safely be sure that she ovulates the same time each month. The time of ovulation will be marked on the temperature chart by a lowering of the temperature followed by a twelve to twenty-four hour elevation of temperature to about 99.4° to 99.6°. The trouble with this method is that even in those women who ovulate regularly at a certain time, under special circumstances—such as an illness, an emotional shock, or recent travel from one place to another—ovulation may shift by two to three days. Generally it has been the custom to refrain from intercourse for about three days before the suspected date of ovulation and three days after the suspected date of ovulation. However, as one can easily see this is not a very scientific method.

BIRTH CONTROL PILLS

A number of birth control pills have come upon the market, and this makes it extremely difficult for both the physician and the patient to choose. The birth control pill is composed of hormones, usually a mixture of estrogen and progesterone hormones that are normally made by the female. A slightly larger amount than is usually secreted in one day is given. When the first pills came out they were in strong doses and caused a lot of symptoms, such as retention of fluid, headaches, changes in personality, and sometimes nausea. (Some of these symptoms are identical with the symptoms of pregnancy in the first three months.) Fortunately, today many of the drug companies have produced a pill with a very low dosage, so that many of the side effects have been eliminated. However, the pills that were initially marketed caused less breakthrough bleeding and less persistent bleeding during the menses than do the newer ones. The pills with the lower dosage are more frequently associated with breakthrough bleeding. Yet, all in all, these pills are much safer than any of the other contraceptive methods that I have mentioned so far. They are about ninety-nine percent effective or better.

A lot of women have read reports in the newspaper and other news media that have warned about the complications of the pill, such as optic neuritis, phlebitis (inflammation of the veins), pulmonary embolism (clots going to the lung), and the possibility of cancer. I feel these reports are exaggerated and should not deter anyone from using the pill if she feels that she needs it for population control or economic reasons. Pregnancy can lead to the same complications as exist with the pill, and in addition the woman runs other risks of childbirth, which are not inherent in the pill. A pregnant woman can develop toxemia or severe bleeding—indeed, she might bleed to death. She can develop phlebitis in the legs and heavy varicose veins. She runs the risk of infection every time she has a child. None of these complications are nearly as frequent in women using the pill, and certainly a woman using the pill would never die of infection or severe bleeding, except under the most peculiar circumstances. A major advantage of the pill is the fact that lovemaking can proceed in a normal, natural fashion without any fear.

One of the disadvantages of the pill is the fact that the woman must remember to take it every night, because if she misses one day she may have breakthrough bleeding, and there may (rarely) be ovulation. A few women get side effects, such as depression, nausea, and retention of fluid. For the male there are none of these disadvantages. Recently an injection has come out that can be given once every four to five months to prevent ovulation. This may gain wider reception because it eliminates taking a pill every day; also, because periods are stopped for months! There is a psychological disadvantage of taking the pill. Many women prior to using the pill were able to resist their husband on the basis that they feared pregnancy, or because they did not have a contraceptive device handy. Now they cannot use this excuse for not giving in to their husbands' desires. Women who use the pills should have "Pap" smears at least every six months to observe for cervicitis or cancer, although it is doubtful that the pills cause either of these.

In summary, I would recommend the pill as the ideal contraceptive device for those women who absolutely cannot have children at the moment. However, for married couples who have had a couple of children and would not be extremely upset if they had a third child, I feel the IUD is the most satisfactory means of contraception. When a woman has had three or more children and is over thirty-five years of age, sterilization by laproscopy (page 318) is the procedure of choice.

ABORTION

What is abortion?

Abortion is the spontaneous or mechanically induced expulsion of an embryo (unborn baby) before the twelfth week of pregnancy. Spontaneous abortions may occur as often as one for every four live births. This means at least one million occur each year in the United States alone. Now that legal abortions can be obtained the figure for abortions will no doubt double or triple.

What causes it?

Spontaneous abortions most frequently occur because of defective germ plasma. This means that if the abortion didn't occur the baby would be born with several defects anyway. So the spontaneous abortion is nature's way of protecting us. Some abortions occur as a result of a hormone imbalance in the mother or certain deformities of the womb. Today many abortions are mechanically induced by physicians.

Who should have a therapeutic abortion?

This is controversial, but I want to make my opinion clear. Therapeutic abortion to me is just one form of contraception.

I do not believe that the embryo before it can survive outside the body is a spiritual entity or human being. It must reach at least the fifth month before it could survive outside the mother. Therefore induced abortion prior to that time is not murder, any more than using contraceptives to kill the sperm or the eggs is. Any unmarried woman should be entitled to have abortion on demand. Married women should be entitled to have an abortion with the written consent of their husbands. The risk of abortion performed in a sterile environment by a licensed physician is minimal. A physician I know who recently passed away did fifty thousand abortions with only one maternal death, and that was because the woman failed to report an infection.

To me the recent Supreme Court decision was a godsend. For example, why should a woman who has been raped have to carry a criminal's child? Why should a daughter have to carry her father's child? These and many more problems with far-reaching psychological and social ramifications have been cleared up by this decision.

Cortisone

What is cortisone?

Cortisone is a hormone secreted by the adrenal gland, particularly the cortex of the adrenal gland, which is useful in the treatment of numerous diseases. This hormone, next to penicillin, has been the most remarkable discovery for the treatment of diseases in our century. There are many analogues to cortisone, such as prednisone, Decadron, Aristocort, but all of these drugs have the same effects, except with greater or lesser potency. In addition the new analogues have been developed to avoid the toxic side effects of cortisone.

What does it do?

Cortisone, whether it is taken orally, intravenously, intramuscularly, or applied locally to the affected site in the body, reduces inflammation, reduces allergy to substances, and even reduces temperature in systemic elements. In short, it cuts down on the body's reaction to disease. In conditions such as allergies or chronic inflammatory conditions of unknown causes, such as rheumatoid arthritis, it is valuable for cutting down on inflammatory responses of the body. However, in infectious diseases it may not be as valuable because it allows the organism to invade the body without resistance.

What is cortisone used for?

Cortisone is used for a variety of disorders. While it was first used in rheumatoid arthritis, it is becoming extremely useful in asthma, hay fever, rheumatic fever, ulcerative colitis, certain forms of meningitis, glomerulonephritis, many chronic joint diseases, and, probably most important, in many chronic skin diseases and allergies. Outside of antibiotics, it is the most frequently prescribed drug today.

Is it dangerous?

Cortisone is potentially a very dangerous drug. It can cause ulcerations in the intestinal tract; it can cause high blood pressure; it can lower resistance to infections such as tuberculosis, etc.; it may cause loss of calcium from the bone and weakening of the bones; it can cause severe depression; it may cause acne of the skin; and it can cause obesity. There are numerous other conditions that it may cause. It delays healing, so that a person who has been on cortisone for a long time may have a difficult period of convalescence following surgery.

What can we do about these side effects?

The most important thing is to prevent them. That is why today cortisone is usually given in short courses. If cortisone is given for a week or less it is rarely associated with any of these toxic effects. I use cortisone frequently in my practice for short courses of a week or less. It is only when cortisone is used over two or three weeks or more that it begins to lead to these toxic effects. When I have to give cortisone over a long period of time there are two ways that I can give it to eliminate these potent side effects. The first way is to give it on alternate days, prescribing three or four tablets every other morning, for example. The second way is to give cortisone for four to five days and interrupt it for two to three days, then begin the same procedure over again. In this way I have been able to use cortisone in rheumatoid arthritis, asthma, and many other chronic conditions without any potent side effects.

D and C

What is a D and C?

A D and C is a dilation and curettage (scraping) of the womb. The cervix is dilated and the lining of the womb is scraped off so that a new and more uniform lining can grow.

Why must I have a D and C?

The most common reason for performing a D and C is because of *dysfunctional vaginal bleeding,* that is, bleeding that does not occur at the regular time of the period each month, or bleeding that occurs beyond the time of the regular period, or, finally, bleeding that is very heavy during the period and occurs with clots. Of course, your doctor will not recommend a D and C the first and second time you have heavy bleeding or bleeding between your periods. Rather, he may do a few diagnostic tests first or try you on one of the hormones, such as progesterone, to see if he can regulate your cycle; but if the bleeding persists for three, four, or even six months, then he will undoubtedly refer you to a gynecologist or perform a D and C himself. Another common reason for performing a D and C is leaking of blood after a delivery, which may indicate that placental fragments (afterbirth fragments) remain in the womb. After a miscarriage it may be necessary to perform a D and C to get rid of some of the retained parts of the fetus or afterbirth. A D and C is often performed for diagnostic purposes to check for cancer of the womb, a polyp, or to find out if the patient is able to carry children in the womb. Some women who cannot have children find that following a D and C they get pregnant. It is also important to perform a D and C on women who cannot have a period at all.

Is this a dangerous procedure?

No! A D and C is a very simple procedure. In fact it could be performed in a doctor's office. If a woman has a very loose cervix, a curette can be passed easily inside the womb without any pain. However, today most patients are hospitalized for this procedure overnight, simply because it is more convenient to do this under anesthesia. Anesthesia has very little danger today. However, your doctor may discharge you before the results of your D and C are back from the pathology lab. Do not get on pins and needles wondering whether you have cancer, because only a few who have a D and C show up with cancer. Some women get continued spotting following a D and C, and therefore it may be necessary to perform a second D and C to relieve the bleeding. This is not a very frequent occurrence.

How many D and C's can you have?

You can have them as frequently as your doctor or a qualified obstetrician and gynecologist feels it is necessary. If the bleeding does not stop after repeated D and C's then a hysterectomy may be necessary. Do not spend time arguing with your doctor whether you need it or not. He knows best!

Digitalis

What is digitalis?

Digitalis is an extract of the beautiful foxglove plant, flowering biennial indigenous to many parts of the United States. This extract is compounded in the form of pills and liquid and administered to patients with heart disease. It exerts a useful effect on heart muscle.

What does it do?

Digitalis increases the contractility and the effectiveness of contraction of the heart muscle, particularly in patients with congestive heart failure. It often slows the heart rate, and in addition it increases the cardiac output. It also has a diuretic action, but this is not major except in patients with heart disease. Digitalis also prevents the development of extra beats and other arrhythmias in patients with heart failure.

What is it used for?

Digitalis is given to patients with congestive heart failure, in other words, people who have fluid accumulation in the lungs or the legs because the heart does not contract either fully or effectively enough. This is the major reason for prescribing digitalis. Many of your friends may have heart failure. The heart failure may be the result of many different diseases, but it will respond to digitalis regardless, as long as it is not due to a major defect.

Digitalis is also prescribed for many irregularities in the heart beat, such as extra systoles (contractile beats), auricular tachycardias (too-rapid heartbeat), and auricular fibrillation (rapid, irregular heartbeat).

Is it dangerous?

Yes. Digitalis if given in large doses can be dangerous. This is why it must be taken only under the supervision of your physician. Side effects, such as nausea and vomiting and other gastrointestinal effects, are not a big problem; it is when it affects the heart that digitalis becomes a real danger. Digitalis may induce the very irregularities in the heart beat that it is prescribed to stop. Therefore, it may cause auricular fibrillation and ventricular tachycardia or auricular flutter and many other disorders of the heart.

Narcotics

What are narcotics?

Narcotics are a group of drugs, usually made from opium, that blunt the mind and when used constantly cause addiction. The most commonly prescribed narcotics are codeine, Demerol, morphine, and Dilaudid. Several synthetic narcotics have been made that are not as addicting; Darvon, Talwin, and Ponstel are just a few. Narcotic addicts use heroin most commonly.

What are they used for?

These drugs are the best things we have to relieve severe or persistent pain. However, they should not be used unless other drugs, such as aspirin, have been unsuccessful or unless a simultaneous investigation is being made to find the cause of the pain. This is because they can be addicting after prolonged use. Morphine is also useful in congestive heart failure (page 180); it sedates the patient and may have a direct effect on eliminating fluid from the lungs. I do not worry about using narcotics frequently in incurable and terminal illness such as cancer. Relief of pain is important enough here to outweigh the disadvantages of making someone an addict. But the correct diagnosis must be established before this position can be assumed.

Are they dangerous?

Yes! The main danger of narcotics is addiction (page 210). Even the milder synthetic narcotics such as Darvon can be addicting. In large enough doses these drugs can suppress the nervous system and respirations and cause death. Allergic reactions and sensitivity are infrequent. Narcotics should be administered only under your physician's supervision.

Penicillin and Antibiotics

What are penicillin and antibiotics?

Antibiotics are drugs that kill or inhibit the growth of microorganisms. Penicillin was one of the first ever discovered, but now there are over fifty different antibiotics and hundreds of preparations on the market. These drugs are the miracle of the twentieth century. They have saved millions of lives in the past thirty years. Other antibiotics that have been discovered since penicillin are the tetracyclines, chloramphenicol, furadantin, neomycin, colymycin, and a host of synthetic penicillins. Most of these were made originally from molds.

What are they used for?

Antibiotics are used to fight bacterial infections in all parts of the body. They have cured millions of cases of pneumonia. They have cured a similar number of ear infections and saved many children's hearing. They wipe out kidney infections, venereal disease and skin infections. They are not useful against most viruses, but they have cured many cases of trachoma, a virus of the eye, and kept many people from going blind. A few antibiotics, such as mycostatin and amphotericin-B, are useful against fungi (molds), the very organisms that antibiotics are made from.

Are they dangerous?

Yes, if used improperly. Every year a few people die from penicillin allergy. All antibiotics can cause death from an allergic reaction. Usually people who are allergic to antibiotics develop a skin rash or asthmatic reaction. Fortunately only a few people are allergic to them. Many of the drugs have toxic effects. For example Chloromycetin may cause a severe anemia. Streptomycin may cause loss of hearing. Keflin and sulfa may cause "blockage" of the kidneys. Macrodantin may cause severe nausea and vomiting. For these and other reasons you should never insist on taking an antibiotic when your doctor says *No!* So many infections seen today are due to a virus that will not be killed by the antibiotic anyway. Your doctor knows best.

Physiotherapy

What is physiotherapy?

Physiotherapy is the treatment of diseases or bodily defects by physical remedies and exercises. It is an extremely important method of medical treatment. There are five common types of physiotherapy: exercise, massage, heat, traction, and physical reconditioning.

Who needs physiotherapy?

Everyone could benefit from physiotherapy. Regular daily exercise and building up of muscle groups that we use most in our daily occupations are extremely valuable. Patients with diseases of the nervous system, however, benefit most from physiotherapy and are the ones most commonly treated. Patients with strokes paralysing one side of the body need active and passive exercises early, and later they need retraining of the paralyzed part. Patients with sprained backs need certain exercises, deep heat or ultrasound (high frequency sound waves) and diathermy (production of heat by electric currents). Patients with bursitis and muscle pains anywhere can also benefit from deep heat and exercise. Patients with slipped discs of the neck or back often benefit from traction and ultrasound. Polio victims need reconditioning and retraining of their legs for walking, etc. Amputees need retraining with an artificial limb.

Is it dangerous?

When performed by a registered physiotherapist, physiotherapy can do no harm and will improve most conditions for which it is prescribed. Even manipulation by a chiropractor can help if there is no serious underlying condition. However, you should always see your physician to establish the correct diagnosis before you visit a chiropractor.

Psychotherapy

What is psychotherapy?

Psychotherapy is the treatment of diseases of the mind and emotions with psychiatric techniques. We usually separate drug therapy of the mind and emotions (psychotherapeutics) from treatment by spending time with a psychiatrist or other doctor to discuss your emotional problems. In group psychotherapy the emotional problems are discussed with other psychiatric patients under the direction of a trained psychotherapist. The simplest form of psychotherapy is discussing an emotional problem with your physician. Just having an understanding listener is good psychotherapy; knowing someone else is concerned about you may boost your ego enough to get you through. Your friend or relative could perform this function if he did not become too emotionally involved and start giving advice.

There are two important rules for the psychotherapist to follow in general: don't give advice and don't become emotionally involved with the patient. The psychotherapist usually serves merely as a guide to the patient through his conscious and subconscious conflicts. In actual practice, however, there are occasions when advice should be given and patients need to see the emotional reaction of the therapist. Many general practitioners, because of their long relationship with the patient, are in a good position to give advice on simple problems. For example, a young college girl nineteen years old has fallen in love with a young college boy and, after a two-month courtship, wants to get married. She asks her family doctor's opinion. He gives quick and considerate advice: wait another three to four months until you know him better.

More intensive psychotherapy is called psychoanalytically oriented psychotherapy. In this form of therapy there is an attempt to solve an acute or subacute anxiety or depressive reaction by trying to find the cause. Many of these conditions can be cured by finding the subconscious factor that underlies them. Sometimes this can be correlated to something that happened during early childhood development. If the patient wants only to resolve this issue, no attempt is made to completely reorganize or reconstruct the personality. The therapist merely aims to cure the anxiety, depression, phobia or hysteria in as simple a way as possible. This form of therapy may take one to two hours a week for up to sixteen weeks, but rarely longer. In this form of therapy the patient may develop a "transference," which means that he or she relates to the therapist as a "father," "brother," "lover," etc. A patient's "love" for the therapist makes him want to get better. Often this transference is subconscious, and the therapist would not try to expose or interpret it unless he wanted to progress to more prolonged and intensive therapy.

In longer term psychotherapy and psychoanalysis, the "transference" is usually exposed so that the patient will be able to understand himself better. This form of therapy may take two to five years. The personality is reorganized and integrated; unrealistic defenses are eliminated; and the system is purged of subconscious anxiety-producing conflicts. Subconscious hostility and guilt are exposed. The patient achieves the goal of "know thyself." Everyone could benefit from this form of therapy, but few have the time or money to do it. Even if we did there wouldn't be enough analysts to do it.

Who should have psychotherapy?

Almost everyone could benefit somewhat from psychotherapy. We all undergo anxiety and depression at certain periods in our lives. It is only when the anxiety or depression persists longer than a few weeks that we need to seek professional help. Actually only a few people are properly motivated to benefit significantly from long-term therapy. An understanding talk with their physician and gentle reassurance is all most people with emotional problems need to get over their condition. Patients who have a mental disturbance (psychosis) cannot benefit very much from psychotherapy. Indeed, psychoanalysis is contraindicated in severe schizophrenia.

Is psychotherapy dangerous?

If performed by an unqualified person it could be. A doctor who doesn't know how to handle the transference may suddenly become involved in a situation he can't handle. For example, if he responds physically in a "lover"-type transference he may cause the patient considerable guilt or interrupt treatment at a very important point. Psychotherapy may bring repressed suicidal ideas to the conscious, and some patients will carry them out.

Hypnosis

This form of treatment has diagnostic and therapeutic value, although limited. In the hypnotic state the patient may reveal subconscious guilt, hostility, and other conflicts that can subsequently be applied in conscious psychotherapy. During hypnosis the psychotherapist can make suggestions that will eliminate certain neuroses. For instance, a therapist may suggest that alcohol or cigarettes should not be indulged in. Unfortunately, while the hypnosis may remove these bad habits, other bad habits may take their place because the therapist has not removed the cause, specifically the anxiety or hostility, that caused them in the first place.

Shots

Many patients have the misconception that a shot or injection of penicillin or some other substance will cure them much faster that any drug taken by mouth. In most cases this is not true. I have had so many patients come to me and ask me for a shot for their cold. If indeed they do have an ordinary common cold, a shot of penicillin or any other antibiotic or any other substance isn't going to do them much good. That is because the common cold is caused by a virus, and it cannot be destroyed by any shot. Of course, there are adenovirus vaccines and influenza vaccine that can prevent some of the cold viruses from developing. These you must take before you get the cold.

Then there are other conditions that people believe a shot will cure. But in reality it doesn't do too much good other than to soothe the anxiety. Shots of B_{12} for severe nerves are not often a very effective method of treating nervous conditions, particularly if that is the only treatment. You will find that a shot of B_{12} along with added anti-depressants or tranquilizers may be an effective treatment. The only condition that B_{12} definitely cures is pernicious anemia, and very few people with nervous conditions have this.

Vitamin shots are not usually any more effective than taking vitamins by mouth. We are fortunate today that so many of the antibiotics can be given by mouth. Occasionally a shot of penicillin is the best way to cure the condition; an example of this is syphilis. And occasionally with subacute bacterial endocarditis or a streptococcal infection of the valves of the heart, penicillin should be given intravenously. But usually if you are coming to the doctor's office and you are able to walk, a pill can be given by mouth and is just as effective to cure your bacterial infection.

Sterilization

What is sterilization?

Sterilization is a form of contraception. In the male, the surgical procedure is called vasectomy. In the female, the surgical procedure is called a tubal ligation.

How is it performed?

A vasectomy can be done under local anesthesia in a doctor's office or the hospital outpatient clinic. After carefully washing the scrotum (the sac that holds the testicles), a little Novocain is injected into the scrotum just at the area of the vas deferens (the tubes that carry the sperm from the testicles to the penis). Then an incision is made over each vas deferens and they are exposed, ligated with catgut or other suture material, and cut. Then the incisions are sewed up with one or two sutures. The whole procedure takes less than half an hour.

A tubal ligation may be performed in two ways now. The old conventional method was to make a four- to five-inch incision over the lower abdomen and enter the abdominal cavity and grab each tube (actually the oviducts that bring the egg-sac to the womb), ligate it with suture material and cut it. This was usually performed under general anesthesia and took forty-five minutes to an hour. In the last few years tubal ligation by laproscopy has become popular. This is sometimes called the "Band-Aid" operation, because the two incisions are so small they can be covered by two Band-Aids. The laproscope is a metal tube with a lens and a light at the end so one can see into the abdomen through a very small incision. Under local or general anesthesia, a half-inch incision is made at the belly button; and after filling the belly with harmless carbon dioxide gas so that the abdominal wall won't hide the organs, the laproscope is inserted through the incision. The tubes are located and then a slender forceps is passed through a second small incision and each tube is grasped and cauterized (burned). The whole procedure takes less than half an hour. But the real beauty of the operation is that there is no unsightly scar to remind the woman of her sterility.

Who should have sterilization performed?

This is a matter of opinion and religious conviction. Any woman or man with a strong hereditary predilection for a life-threatening or crippling disease (severe mental retardation, etc.) should probably have this done if he or she wants to get married. Parents in this position can successfully adopt children and fulfill their maternal or paternal instincts. I personally believe that women with four children should definitely have this procedure done and women who desire it after two children should be allowed to have it done. Men should not have a vasectomy until after fifty-five or sixty because it seems to affect their ego more and may cause inflammation of the testicles severe enough to cause impotence. There are reports that vasectomies may predispose to other diseases.

Is it dangerous?

The procedure itself is not dangerous. The operation is short, anesthesia local, and the surgeon is not attacking vital organs. The long-term psychological effects will depend on the person involved. As I said above, a vasectomy may lead to other medical problems.

Tonsillectomy

What is a tonsillectomy?

A tonsillectomy is the removal of two large lymph glands that lie at the back of the throat, just above the tongue, in what we call the pharyngeal cavity. A lot of work has been done to prove that the tonsils harbor diseases of all kinds and contribute to many diseases. However, very few of these reports can be well substantiated. Therefore, the wholesale removal of tonsils that was occurring up until the past two decades was not warranted. It is true that before the antibiotic age, tonsils were a consistent source of streptococcal infections, which as you probably know, contribute to rheumatic fever and nephritis. Now that antibiotics are available, particularly prophylactic penicillin for the rheumatic fever victim, it seems unwarranted to remove the tonsils even in these patients. The main indications for a tonsillectomy are obstruction to swallowing and/or breathing and recurrent ear infections. A tonsillectomy usually includes removal of the adenoids, which are lymphoid tissues at the back of the nose just above the throat. These are also responsible for difficulty in breathing. There can be no doubt that people who have obstruction of the nasal passages by large adenoids or by tonsils have less incidence of colds or throat ailments after removal of these organs. Ear infections are also very frequent in people with large tonsils and adenoids.

What is the operation like?

This is usually a very simple operation. It is performed under local anesthesia in a large number of patients, but in younger children it is better performed under general anesthesia. After the patient is anesthetized, an instrument with a large loop of wire that can be contracted is placed around the tonsil and then this is closed and contracted and the tonsil pinched off. Usually there is very little postoperative bleeding, but on occasion this can be massive. This is why the doctor keeps the patient in the hospital overnight after the removal of the tonsils. After coming out of the anesthesia the patient feels as if he has swallowed a football, but this gradually wears off over the next two or three days. Most patients can take broth and juices within a couple of hours after the operation. There are throat lozenges available today that almost completely anesthetize the area to keep the pain down to a minimum.

Tranquilizers

Tranquilizers are a group of drugs used to treat anxiety, depression, and severe mental diseases such as schizophrenia. Next to the antibiotics (penicillin, etc.) and steroid drugs (cortisone, etc.), they are the most important group of drugs to be discovered in the twentieth century. Millions of people have been released from the state mental institutions because of these drugs. Millions of others live productive, orderly, and carefree lives because of them. Probably the first drug to be used as a tranquilizer was phenobarbital. This is very useful for anxiety and tension. Today Librium and Valium are used just as frequently for anxiety and tension as phenobarbital.

Thorazine (a phenothiazine) was probably the first drug to be labeled a "tranquilizer" and deserves the distinction of causing a revolution in the treatment of severe mental diseases. Before Thorazine these conditions were treated with rest, institutionalization, and insulin, or electro-shock therapy. Now shock treatment and institutionalization are rarely necessary. Many relatives of Thorazine have been developed, but they all work basically the same way and none has replaced Thorazine completely. In the past decade many tranquilizers have been developed to fight depression, such as Elavil and Sinequan. These are extremely useful and prevent a lot of people from committing suicide. We are very lucky to live in the era of such miraculous drugs.

Narcotics (page 310) should not be considered tranquilizers, but unfortunately they are often used as such.

Vaccination

What is a vaccine?

A vaccine is a substance made up of dead bacteria or viruses, or partially killed bacteria or viruses, which is made into an emulsion and injected into the human being to produce immunity against these infectious diseases. The vaccine will stimulate antibody formation in the body and thus make antibodies available should actual infection by the disease in question occur. In addition, some vaccines are made of toxins (attenuated toxins). An example of this would be tetanus toxoid. These toxins are ordinarily produced by the bacteria and are almost as harmful or more harmful than the bacteria itself. The most common vaccines used today are tetanus toxoid, pertussis vaccine or whooping cough, diphtheria vaccine, poliomyelitis vaccine, smallpox vaccine, measles vaccine, and mumps vaccine. There are over a hundred different vaccines that are used from time to time in special cases (cholera vaccine, typhoid vaccine, etc.).

What are the recommendations for vaccination of infants and children?

Infants and children generally get the following eight different vaccines: diphtheria, tetanus, whooping cough, poliomyelitis, smallpox, both types of measles, and mumps vaccine. The schedules of administration of these vaccines vary somewhat from doctor to doctor. The following schedule is proposed by the American Academy of Pediatrics. The diphtheria, tetanus, and whooping cough vaccines are administered between two and six months of age, and a poliomyelitis vaccine is administered at two months of age. Then the ordinary measles vaccine can be given at nine months, and a smallpox vaccine can be given anywhere from six to twelve months of age. The German measles (rubella) vaccine is often given between one and twelve years of age, or before adolescence. Children with eczema should not receive smallpox vaccine. In fact, the latest thinking in medical circles is that smallpox vaccine should be dispensed with altogether, unless an epidemic is forthcoming.

What are the recommended vaccines for adults?

Adults who have not had poliomyelitis vaccine should get one immediately. Also, adults who have not had tetanus vaccine should get two successive shots about one month apart to be adequately immunized. Adult males who have not had mumps should get the mumps vaccine. Adult females who have not had German measles and who are sufficiently warned about the possibilities of pregnancy and are taking contraceptives to avoid it can be given the German measles vaccine. There must be complete certainty that pregnancy cannot occur during the period of establishing immunization with this vaccine. No adult who has not had smallpox vaccine need at the present time get a smallpox vaccine unless he is traveling outside of the country.

Other vaccines are recommended under special circumstances. Generally, typhoid vaccines are given when one is under the risk of being exposed to typhoid, such as in foreign countries. Tuberculosis vaccines are not generally given unless people are working with tuberculous patients. The same goes for leprosy vaccine. Rabies vaccine is usually not given unless after a ten- to fourteen-day period of observation the suspected dog actually develops rabies. If the dog develops rabies then the human who has been bitten is given rabies vaccine. One in three thousand people develop allergic encephalitis from this vaccine, so therefore it is not used unless the dog is certain to have rabies.

If I have never received any of the vaccinations, can I be vaccinated when I get a particular infection?

Generally vaccines are of no help once the infection has actually begun, although there are some exceptions to this rule. However, your doctor may inject you with another immunizing substance to fight disease. This is usually passive immunization in the form of an antiserum. The antisera are made from injecting vaccine into animals or by actually infecting the animal with a bacteria or virus. Then the animal's blood is drained of its antibodies in the form of a serum. Thus, if you get bitten and have not had tetanus toxoid, you can receive tetanus antitoxin, which can be from horse, cattle, or from human serum. The same type of immunity can be given to you if you happen to contract diphtheria or pertussis, but it is not as effective.

What are the recommendations for immunization for travel?

All countries have varying vaccination requirements, depending upon what infectious diseases are prominent in their area. However, any traveler who leaves the United States must have had a successful vaccination against smallpox within three years prior to re-entry to the United States, or prior to leaving the United States if he is returning within a short period. These vaccinations are both for your welfare and for the welfare of all the people whom you may be exposed to once you re-enter the United States, because you could act as a carrier of the disease. Many countries have vaccination requirements for typhoid, cholera, diphtheria, plague, polio, tetanus, typhus, etc. To list all these would be foolish. However, your doctor will know what vaccination requirements are needed according to the itinerary of your trip.

Vitamins

What are vitamins?

Vitamins are a group of chemical compounds that are essential to body metabolism but cannot be produced by the body and must therefore be supplied in the diet. Likewise, there are certain unsaturated fats and amino acids that are just as essential to the body and must be supplied by the diet. Yet, the vitamins as you know them and as we physicians prescribe are vitamin A, the B vitamins, vitamin C or ascorbic acid, vitamins D, and E, and K. The vitamins actually are divided into two groups according to whether they are fat-soluble or water-soluble. Water-soluble vitamins are the B group of vitamins. These include thiamine, niacin, pyridoxine, riboflavin, and B_{12} or cyanocobalamin. The rest are fat-soluble.

Vitamins are put on the market in three different ways. They can be bought as the specific vitamin, such as vitamin A, vitamin D, thiamine or nicotinic acid, separately. Or you can buy a multiple vitamin, which would contain all the vitamins in the minimum daily requirement and would therefore be a vitamin for prophylaxis of vitamin deficiencies, or what we call a maintenance vitamin. Or you can buy a therapeutic vitamin, which would include one or all of the essential vitamins in much larger doses than the minimum daily requirement, sometimes ten to fifteen times above the minimum daily requirement.

Actually, overt vitamin deficiencies are rare in our Western civilization, because most of the vitamins can be partially supplied by an adequate and balanced diet. On the other hand, subclinical vitamin deficiencies are probably common in our society, first of all, because none of us are dietitians and cannot plan our diets perfectly; secondly, because we eat out in restaurants, where the vitamins are often steamed out of the food; and finally, we often choose what we eat on the basis of our taste and not on the basis of whether it is good for us or not. The deficiencies of vitamin A, D, and even C are rare in adults and rarely show clinical symptoms, because vitamin D is supplied in milk and C is supplied in orange juice and most green leafy vegetables contain an adequate amount of vitamin A for our diets. However, alcoholics frequently are deficient in the B vitamins. In older adults a disease called pernicious anemia, which is due to the deficiency of vitamin B_{12}, is often seen due to premature atrophy of the gastric mucosa. Occasionally this is seen in younger people due to a hereditary deficiency of a factor secreted by the lining of the stomach. The lining of the stomach produces a substance called the intrinsic factor, which is necessary for the absorption of B_{12} from food. Thus pernicious anemia is not due to lack of B_{12} in the diet in most cases but it is more frequently due to a lack of the intrinsic factor, preventing B_{12} from being absorbed.

What are the symptoms and signs of vitamin deficiencies?

Vitamin A deficiency usually produces thickening of the cornea, night blindness and eventually day blindness, and dry skin and rashes. There is no label for this disease other than vitamin A deficiency. A deficiency of the B vitamins is divided into three basic types clinically. One is deficiency of B_1 (thiamine) and it is called beri-beri. This is manifested by swelling of the legs and puffiness of the body, as well as paralysis in some cases of the arms and legs, enlargement of the heart, and shortness of breath. Deficiency of niacin usually produces a clinical syndrome called pellagra, in which there are skin rashes, neuritis causing paralysis of the hands or feet, and diarrhea due to intestinal involvement; mental deterioration, such as forgetfulness and delerium, may occur due to central nervous system involvement. Riboflavin deficiency causes "perleche," in which the corners of the mouth break, and often dimness and blurring of vision with sensitivity to light. In children pyridoxine deficiency (vitamin B_6) may lead to convulsions. This has not been labeled by a certain name. Vitamin C deficiency is manifested clinically by scurvy, in which there are hemorrhages of the gums, joints, and sometimes hemorrhages of the skin and poor teeth. Vitamin D deficiency is manifested by rickets or osteomalacia, in which there is softening of the bone due to loss of calcium, producing bowed legs or knock-knees, etc. Vitamin K deficiency causes bleeding because the blood fails to coagulate well, due to the lack of prothrombin, a substance in the blood that is made from vitamin K; this may cause nosebleeds, gastrointestinal bleeding, blood in the urine, and occasionally bleeding under the skin. These then are the major syndromes that are produced by vitamin deficiencies.

What can I do to prevent vitamin deficiencies?

The best answer would be to eat a well-balanced diet, but since you are not likely to be a dietitian you may have difficulty doing this. I recommend to all my patients that they take a one-a-day vitamin that supplies the minimum daily requirement of each vitamin. This includes at least five thousand units of vitamin A, one thousand units of vitamin D, and seventy-five milligrams of ascorbic acid, as well as one milligram of thiamine, ten milligrams of niacin, one or two milligrams of riboflavin, and one to two milligrams of pyridoxine (vitamin B_6). I don't think it is necessary to take a vitamin that includes B_{12}, and as for the minerals that are often included with these vitamins, most of them are ridiculous.

Fluorine is a valuable supplement in the diet in areas of the country where the drinking water does not supply at least one part per million in the water. This will prevent tooth decay. Sodium, potassium, phosphorus and calcium are usually provided by the foods in the diet. Iron is not always contained in the diet and therefore a one-a-day vitamin with iron makes good sense. This is particularly true in menstruating women between the ages of twelve and forty-five, who require more iron than is supplied in the average diet.

Under certain conditions when a person is subjected to stresses, such as a cold, sore throat or any type of infection, he needs more vitamins. Also when a mother is breast-feeding she needs extra vitamins. When a woman is pregnant she requires extra vitamins, and most women are used to having their obstetrician or family physician supply them with vitamins during pregnancy. Infants who are breast-fed need supplements of certain vitamins, and most pediatricians prescribe some sort of vitamin to all children before they are able to consume the ordinary diet. A lot of the formulas have vitamins and iron added to them, and this is a good idea. People who have false teeth or who can't chew their food well should take a vitamin, without any question. People dieting should take a vitamin, because this will help burn the fat and protein that is being released by the breakdown of the tissues. When a patient is on prolonged bed rest in a hospital it is often valuable to take a vitamin supplement. These are just a few of the special circumstances when a vitamin is extremely valuable for prophylaxis as well as therapy.

Are vitamins dangerous?

If a patient took an excess amount of the multiple vitamin capsules every day he would certainly not get any toxic effects from the vitamin B's. It has never been proved that any of the B group will cause toxic effects. Large doses of ascorbic acid have never been proved to be harmful. However, to take a thousand milligrams or more a day for a cold has never been proved to be effective, despite recent reports. Excessive amounts of vitamin E have never caused any problems either. Excessive amounts of vitamin A, particularly in infants, can cause hyperostosis of the bones, weight loss, cracking and bleeding of the lips, fatigue, abdominal discomfort, and bone and joint pain. Excessive amounts of vitamin D can cause increased calcium both in the tissues and the kidneys, leading to renal stones, and there may be symptoms of nausea, vomiting, diarrhea and headache. Excessive amounts of vitamin K may be dangerous in newborn infants. So, in summary, one may take large amounts of the B vitamins, such as thiamine, nicotinic acid, riboflavin, and pyridoxine, without any harmful effects, but vitamins A, D, and K should never be taken in large amounts for a prolonged period of time.

Water Pills

I have so frequently had patients come to me and ask for water pills for getting rid of fluid that I think a discussion of this subject is appropriate. Water pills, or diuretics, are really pills that get rid of the salt in our system. To a certain extent a large amount of water will go out with the salt. Water pills should be given only to people who have an excess of salt in their system and cannot get rid of it by normal means. There are an awful lot of obese people and people with varicose veins who appear to have extra fluid in their systems but in reality do not. It is just that the fluid is in a different place. Most of these water pills act on the kidney to prevent the reabsorption of salt or to help secrete larger amounts of salt. They are given to people with congestive heart failure, chronic liver disease, or chronic kidney disease. Occasionally they may be given to someone who is extremely overweight for the psychological value of getting rid of five to ten pounds in the first twenty-four hour period of dieting.

However, these pills are not without side effects. For instance, they may cause an excessive loss of potassium salts rather than sodium salts from the body and in this way lead to weakness, fatigue, a distended bowel, and mental confusion. Also, their prolonged use can cause damage to the kidneys. They may cause an elevated blood sugar and uric acid (the acid that causes gout). They can also cause occasional kidney stones in susceptible people. Patients should therefore not put undue pressure on their physicians to prescribe these drugs unless there is a sound medical reason.

X-Ray Therapy

It is well known to the layman that the use of x-ray in the treatment of cancers of various organs has become extremely valuable. In some cases we are able to completely wipe out the tumor by x-ray therapy alone. The doses of x-ray given in x-ray therapy are much greater than those used in diagnosis (i.e., taking x-ray pictures). Cancers of the skin can be completely wiped out by x-ray. Cancers of the uterus can be completely wiped out by x-ray treatment. The use of x-ray will slow down the progress of certain cancers and sometimes hold them at bay for a long time. For example, x-ray treatment of a lung tumor may slow it down considerably. However, there are some tumors that do not respond to x-ray therapy, such as tumors of the bone, muscle, and stomach. Since there is a variability of response to x-ray treatment, patients should not be surprised if their doctor does not refer them for x-ray treatment. In some cases your doctor will make a last-ditch stand against the tumor by trying x-ray. X-ray treatment is not very toxic and many people experience no symptoms at all after a treatment. Others get nausea and vomiting and their skin may break out in severe rash. The postradiation upset of the stomach usually only lasts a few days. X-rays also may damage the ovaries or testes and prevent reproduction. In our huge cobalt units today more highly intense x-ray may be administered to smaller areas so that adverse reactions to x-ray are much less frequent. X-ray treatment is used most often in conjunction with surgery. However, it may be the sole treatment for some tumors.

HOME HEALTH CARE

Health Tips

Many patients have asked me how they can live a healthy life and exactly what they should do to prevent themselves from getting serious illnesses. I feel that the care of the body can be divided into various categories.

Diet

First of all, it is very important that you have a well-balanced diet. The size of the diet may vary, depending upon what kind of occupation you have. If you are a laborer who has to do a lot of heavy lifting and vigorous work, then you may need 3500 to 4000 calories, but if your work is mainly sedentary then 800 to 2000 calories may be perfectly adequate. The quality of the diet should include the basic seven: (1) meat, fish, or eggs; (2) milk or milk products; (3) green and yellow vegetables, (4) fruit, (5) whole-grain bread or cereals; (6) starchy vegetable; and (7) butter or margarine. What is needed most are certain unsaturated fats that cannot be produced by the body, a good allotment of vitamins, and the essential amino acids.

To prevent too much intake of cholesterol one should follow these six basic suggestions:

1. No more than two eggs per week.
2. Switch from butter to margarine.
3. Cut all visible fat off your meat.
4. Restrict gravy.
5. Broil all meat.
6. Take grease from food. Use vegetable oils to cook. Vegetable oils contain very little cholesterol.

It's important to have regularity of your meals, but the number of times a person needs to eat during a day may vary with the individual. Of course, our stomach is empty two and one-half hours after a meal, and this may stimulate sending a message from the stomach to the brain of hunger, but whether the body really needs food at that time is another thing. Americans eat too much. Insisting on a big breakfast, a big lunch, and a big supper is pure nonsense. Possibly either a light breakfast or a light lunch should be substituted in this pattern of having three big meals per day. I think it's especially bad to eat a large meal at supper time and then lie down on the couch for a snooze. The food may regurgitate into the esophagus (the tube leading to the stomach) and cause heartburn. On top of that, much of the food is absorbed into the blood stream, creating a high blood fat level, which may lead to a myocardial infarction (heart attack) among other things. If a person goes to bed on a full stomach after a midnight snack, he may not be able to sleep at all. Overeating is almost as bad as drinking or smoking too much. The aim should be everything in moderation and nothing in excess.

Vitamins

It has become common for television commercials to remind you that you need a one-a-day vitamin. I would agree with this concept for the following reasons: first of all, many people eat out and choose from the menu what they want to eat rather than what they should eat. When a person goes to a restaurant he may get food that has been sitting in a hot pan for a number of hours so that many of the vitamins have been steamed out of the food. Second of all, many people today have false teeth or a dental prosthesis and cannot chew food well. Also, not every housewife is a certified dietician and she cannot select the food that is required to get the adequate requirements of vitamins. If possible, a multiple vitamin a day is advisable. If this cannot be achieved, at least twice a week is probably sufficient. True, many foods have vitamins added, such as cereals (Wheaties, etc.) and milk (Vitamin D), but even these foods do not usually contain an adequate amount of vitamins. There is generally no great harm from too many vitamins. If one ingested tremendous amounts of Vitamin D he might develop kidney problems, but this the only disorder I know of in adults that can develop from overdosing with vitamins.

The daily bowel movement

It seems that daily elimination has become an obsession in America. No person feels quite right unless he has moved his bowels at least once a day. This is a real fallacy! Moving the bowels two or three times a week is certainly adequate. A person is not constipated unless he has a very hard stool and moves his bowels less than three times a week. To say that one is constipated simply because he does not move his bowels every day is pure nonsense. Some of my patients have developed a laxative habit, which I abhor. This causes poor absorption of vitamins and other food materials that are necessary for the body, and there are other side effects from some laxatives, which irritate the bowel. Other patients have used enemas every day of their lives. These are not necessary. Only a few of the many people that are using enemas every day need them. If you are going to use enemas because of real constipation, then a low tap water enema should suffice. A Fleets enema might be a good substitute, as it comes already prepared.

Exercise

Americans have become more and more sedentary. Their occupations have shifted from heavy labor to more white collar work. Most of us drive to work now. When we get to work we sit on assembly lines or in an office and do not move anything more than our fingers. Since most of our work is done by machinery, I predict that by the twenty-first century we will have nothing but a large index finger at the end of our arms to push buttons. You can prevent this prediction from coming true if you develop regular daily exercise habits. Not all of us run around the track field or the block daily. It might look a little ridiculous if we all went out in groups and did this. The winter snow might make it pretty difficult. Nor can most of us take time out in a busy day to go swimming at the YMCA or go home to our own pools if we have one. However, exercise by the Canadian Air Force method daily is an excellent way of keeping in shape; this method consists of doing so many sit-ups, so many push-ups, so many jumping jacks, etc., every day. If this is not satisfactory, then I would say you should purchase an exercise cycle. You can get these from $27.00 to $110.00, depending on how much luxury you want. The important thing is to have one with an odometer so that you can tell how far you have gone each day. If you pedal a mile or two every day I think you could keep your heart in shape. You have heard a lot about isometrics, but these are of no value in keeping the heart in shape. If you simply want to build muscles, then weight-lifting and isometric exercises are valuable; but if you want to keep your heart in shape, then isotonic exercises, in which the body muscles are moving through a full range of motion, are the ticket.

Posture

Americans also probably have the worst posture in the world. Many of us slump at our desks. We don't have good backs on our chairs. When we're standing, because of our heights, we bend forward or lean to one side on one foot. I recommend that we be more posture-conscious. Those of us who have had the basic training in the armed forces know what good posture is. But for others it needs to be explained. A person should throw his chest out, shoulders back, head erect and much of the weight should be back on the heels. Sit erect when you're in chairs. We must remind ourselves frequently to do this. I think one of the most useful exercises is hyperextension exercises of the back. This keeps the most important muscles in our body in shape at all times. This can be done by lying flat on a bed and arching the lower part of the back until your hand can go under it without much pressure. Then maintain this hyperextension of the lower back while counting to twenty, release it and perform the same thing over again. If one does this ten minutes in the morning and ten minutes in the evening over a period of two to three weeks, he will find his back muscles will be strong. Assuming correct posture will be a lot easier. It is also important to assume the correct posture when you lift something. We should use the support of our knees when we're lifting something heavy instead of trying to put the whole weight on our backs. It is better to squat down and lift the object with our hands and knees together than to bend at the hips and pick things up with our fingers while our legs remain straight.

Bathing

Americans also bathe too much. Second to overeating this is one of our worst habits. I've known many people who bathe twice a day. They don't feel they are clean unless they do. Here again we are doing something very dangerous to the body, particularly the skin. Our skin becomes macerated (softened and worn), and the natural bacteria are washed away, and deeper layers of our skin are exposed to the weather. The natural oil that keeps our skin in good condition is also removed in this manner. I think two or three baths a week in the winter is sufficient. In the summer no more than one bath a day is needed but preferably one bath every two days. Choice of soap may differ. I have no definite suggestions regarding this. However I have found a lot of people vigorously washing their faces with soap. This should not be performed too vigorously even if you may wish to prevent acne, because you will, again, remove too much of the natural oil and cause irritation of the pores of the skin. The openings of both sweat and sebaceous glands may close over and lead to boils, etc.

Sleep

I'm sure that while Americans get excess food and excess bathing and attempt to move their bowels too much, they generally do not get enough sleep. Most people should get at least eight hours of sleep at night, but this may vary with the individual. Some people may require only four to five hours of sleep a night, while others may require ten hours of sleep each night. We should be careful about standardizing this factor. Forcing our children and ourselves to get a certain number of hours in the pad is important.

It is not necessary to be actually asleep when one lies down and relaxes. If you get eight hours of relaxation a day, I feel that is sufficient whether you are sleeping or not. Some patients become concerned that they're not actually sleeping while they are passing through the night, and they ask for sleeping pills. This is not usually necessary unless a person has a lot on his mind or is suffering from chronic anxiety or depression. If you find it difficult to go to sleep there is nothing wrong with getting up and reading a good relaxing novel or even watching television for a little while. I think one of the reasons that we do not sleep soundly is because we do not exercise adequately, and therefore our muscles are not tired enough to make us feel like sleeping. Yet we are mentally exhausted. There is no harm in taking an occasional sleeping pill if you find that you frequently miss a night of sleep. Like any other pill these can become habit forming. Although this is not the same addiction, dependence on a sleeping pill is liable to increase with each passing day.

A very important point in getting proper sleep is having the proper mattress. I recall that while I was an intern working every third night I used to sleep better at the hospital than at home. This was finally explained by the fact that in the hospital there was a firm mattress, and even though I got only four hours of sleep at the hospital I felt better the next day. When I discovered this we got rid of our old mattress at home and purchased a very firm queen-size mattress, and my wife and I both slept a lot better. The American conception that married couples are not compatible unless they sleep in a double bed is ridiculous. If you are going to have a double bed I would recommend a queen-size or king-size bed. This is especially important when one of the partners is heavier than the other. Invariably the lighter partner finds himself rolling toward the side of the heavier person. There is nothing wrong with twin beds. The sooner we get rid of this hang-up the better.

Sex

Of course for the unmarried people I would like to discuss this problem further under *Marriage* (page 360) and *Premarital Examination* (page 273). For married people I'd say sex varies with the couple. There is nothing unhealthy about sex two to three times a day if both partners are interested in this, but for one person to force himself on the other is ridiculous. The average American couple in their twenties and thirties has intercourse three to four times a week, but in the forties and fifties this gradually dwindles down to once every two weeks and even as low as once a month. What is normal in the frequency of intercourse varies tremendously. The method of intercourse can be as variable as each couple desires, as long as both parties agree.

Vaccinations

I have devoted another section to vaccinations, but in general for good hygiene adults should have at least a tetanus toxoid shot every four years. Smallpox, diphtheria and pertussis vaccine are only necessary for infants and children. In adults smallpox vaccine is necessary if one is going out of the country. I feel the oral polio vaccine should definitely be given to everybody. It is not clear whether a booster dose of this is necessary. At this time it seems unnecessary. Recently measles vaccine has been added to the long list of vaccines available. A mumps vaccine is extremely important for adult males who have never had mumps, because of the high frequency of spread to the testicles with subsequent sterilization. The new rubella (German measles) vaccine should be given to all women who are not pregnant and who have never experienced definite rubella infection in childhood. But this must be given in a cautious fashion, which I will explain subsequently (see page 322).

Care of special organs

In addition to the above health tips, I want to give some health tips regarding special areas of the body. First of all, I think it is absolutely foolish to wash the *hair* more than once a week. I find a lot of my female patients disagree with me. Yet you will remove a lot of the natural oils and may cause a lot more dandruff than you cure if you wash the hair too frequently. Applying special creams to various parts of the body, in my opinion, has done nothing for the *skin,* but I'm sure the cosmetic experts would disagree with me. Care of the *eyes* should involve an eye examination every two years and preferably every year if one is wearing glasses. There have been a lot of eye washes on the market, but it is doubtful that any of these are necessary for the average person unless prescribed by the eye doctor. The same holds for eye drops.

One of the worst things I see in patients is their obsession with digging wax out of the *ears.* This should always be done by a doctor. I would not recommend putting a Q-tip in the ear. The old adage that nothing smaller than your elbow should be put in your ear still holds true, in my opinion. There are a few people who accumulate a tremendous amount of wax, and they should have this washed out by their doctor at periodic intervals.

An examination of the *teeth* with periodic cleaning by a dental hygienist is very basic at least every six months to a year. On top of that, I think use of a toothpaste with fluoride added is very valuable. However, this is not necessary in a community where fluoride is already added to the water. I would suggest that you find out whether fluoride is added to the water in your community, and if not, use fluoride in your toothpaste as well as possibly taking fluoride tablets by mouth periodically. The habit of using *mouth* washes is another ridiculous thing we do. This habit has been caused by the tremendous number of radio and television commercials expounding these products. If you have bad breath it may be worthwhile to use one of these mouth washes, but for daily hygiene it is nonsense. Even when one has a cold or a sore throat these gargles are of no value in getting rid of the infection. You would be better off to gargle with salt water or aspirin.

In general women seem to have an obsession about

douching themselves, particularly after intercourse. This is a very foolish habit! I think the only time a woman should douche is about once a month, following the fifth day of her period. The vagina contains natural bacteria and also an acid pH, which keeps the hygiene excellent in a natural way. To use a vinegar douche more often than once a month only destroys the normal bacteria and may cause other complications. There is nothing dirty about the male semen, and therefore there is no reason to douche after having intercourse with your husband. Of course, if you feel he has been promiscuous or has a venereal disease you should consult your family doctor.

To prevent *varicose veins* I think it is important that women and men who stand on their feet all day wear Supphose or elastic stockings to prevent the veins from dilating. One also should have the proper shoes to insure good posture. Women who wear very high heels with spindle points at the end are only asking for trouble. A lower heel with a good arch and a good fit is best. One may have to go to an orthopedic shoe store to get the proper fit. An ideal shoe would be one that is cast exactly for the foot, but not many of us can afford shoes of this type. If after you have worn a shoe a couple of days you find that it is loose, it would be better to go back and spend the money for a new pair of shoes than to continue to wear a shoe that does not fit adequately. Those of us who have special sizes like triple A, should be fit by an expert.

Although the fingernails should be clipped in a round fashion, the *toenails* must be cut square. If one finds that the side of the nail is turning down into the skin, then a V-shaped wedge should be cut in the center of the nail. This portion may also be filed away if one has difficulty cutting it because of a thick nail. With this procedure there will be fewer ingrown toenails.

Finally, the most important part of good hygiene is a routine *physical examination* at least once a year. For women this includes a "Pap" smear and a breast examination. For men this should include a rectal examination. For both men and women over forty this should include an electrocardiogram, a chest x-ray and certain blood tests. For more discussion on the routine examination, see pages 266-272.

Home Medicine Chest

Many patients ask me what they should have in the home medicine chest. Should a patient treat anything or should he call a doctor for everything he gets? I think it is perfectly justified for a person to treat certain of his own illnesses, which I will mention. He certainly should not treat any of these illnesses if symptoms persist. It is better to call a physician at the first sign of any illness to get his advice over the phone.

The contents of the family medicine chest is a subject of controversy, but for my patients I like to recommend certain things they should keep on hand. Since most of the drugs that you have in your medicine chest presently are old, the first thing you should do is clean the chest out and throw everything outdated away. There are certain things that I feel should *not* be in the medicine chest. These are: tincture of iodine, tincture of merthiolate, old drugs, Vaseline, any non-sterile gauze and bandages, aspirin that does not have a good secure lid on it, Unguentine for burns, any medication for which you do not have a label, and throat gargles. Many of these are worthless and the others are potential dangers if they fall into the hands of children. It would be wise to keep a lock on your medicine chest, although I know this is difficult for most of us.

There is certain general equipment that should be available in the home medicine chest. It should have a bulb syringe for irrigating wounds and the ear. It should have some gauze pads and bandages and one-half-inch and one-inch adhesive tape. Band-Aids should be available. There should be a good eye wash, a thermometer, a heating pad, and an ice pack. There should be a rubber sheet for putting on the bed when a person is suffering from fever, diarrhea that he can't control, or incontinence. A bedpan is also valuable for use when a person is too sick to get out of bed to go to the bathroom. Other than these I would like to discuss drugs and equipment that you should have on hand for the more common illnesses.

Acid indigestion or upset stomach

For this it is wise to have on hand some Maalox or Pepto-Bismol, and if you are traveling it is wise to have tablets of Titralac or Gelusil available. Almost everybody has experienced acid indigestion at one time or another, and there is no reason why the acute cases can't be treated by you. Either the liquid or the tablets should be taken at least every hour or every two hours until good relief is obtained. Of course, if the condition continues longer than twenty-four hours you should consult your physician.

Allergic reactions and hay fever

The layman is capable of treating most mild skin reactions and hay fever, particularly if he knows the cause. For poison ivy, for example, calamine lotion and Pyribenzamine tablets (taken by mouth) are very effective. For children elixir of Benadryl may be given by mouth, as this is a very good antihistamine that will stop itching and cut down on the inflammation in the skin rash. For the more severe allergic reactions, your doctor will prescribe cortisone creams as well as cortisone by mouth or by injection. Hay fever can be treated both by Pyribenzamine tablets and by Neosynephrine nasal spray, as long as the spray is not used too frequently. Dristan and Contact are also helpful in the treatment of nasal allergies. Here again it is important that you know the cause if the condition is persistent or severe.

Colds, influenza, and dry cough

I think one of the most valuable remedies for the cold is *aspirin.* It is an anti-inflammatory agent, bacterial agent, and it helps keep the temperature down and relieves many symptoms of a cold. It can be purchased without a prescription.

In addition, it is wise for you to have an *expectorant* on hand. Benylin or Pertussin and many other cough medicines, such as Vicks-44, may be purchased without a prescription, and these are excellent. If you desire to have an expectorant with codeine in it you must ask your doctor for this. Codeine suppresses a dry cough. In addition nasal and bronchial *decongestants,* such as Actifed tablets or liquid or Ornade (which can be bought only by prescription), might be very valuable. You can get Contact or Dristan, which will serve the same purpose and are available without a prescription.

Vitamin C is valuable to have on hand, but I would not take any more than 100 mg tablets, as more is ridiculous. These can be purchased without a prescription. A *steam vaporizer* should be on hand, and it is nice to use tincture of benzoine with this, which you can get at a drugstore without a prescription. Neosynephrine ¼% is a very valuable nasal spray, which is also available in drops; it is very good for relieving nasal congestion that might otherwise block off the sinuses and cause trouble. Do not use this any more frequently than every four hours. For sore throats along with the cold it is good to have lozenges; Spectrocin-T can be purchased without prescription, as can various other throat lozenges.

Constipation

The treatment of constipation should be within the acumen of any layman. The mildest laxative and the least harmful is milk of magnesia. This can be taken either as tablets or as a liquid according to the directions on the bottle. If you desire something a little more effective, glycerine suppositories or Dulcolax suppositories are very valuable. A Fleets enema sometimes works very well. To prevent constipation mineral oil, one tablespoon daily, may be very valuable. However, your doctor should be consulted if constipation persists, as it may be a sign of definite illness. I find that if a person has an extremely large stool resulting from several days of constipation, it is wise to put K-Y jelly or a similar lubricating material into the rectum before trying to move the bowels. You may also break up the stool with your finger. If one Fleets or tap water enema is ineffective in relieving your constipation, I think your physician should be consulted.

Diarrhea

Every layman should be able to treat acute diarrhea as long as there is no severe temperature associated with it. If there is a large degree of blood or mucus associated with it, then you should consult your doctor. But since most acute diarrheas are due to a viral gastroenteritis, there is no reason why a layman cannot treat it. The most common remedies are Kaopectate and Paregoric. You can ask your physician to give you a prescription for Paregoric to keep on hand. However, it might be wise to have him give you elixir of Donnatal or Lomotil tablets to keep on hand for this problem. It is wise to restrict all your oral intake and take only bouillon or tea and use a hot water bottle on your belly. Some people use Pepto-Bismol and this is corrective in some cases.

Eye trauma, pain, discharge or foreign body

Occasionally you can wipe out a foreign body from your eye with a piece of cotton or the corner of your handkerchief, but you should not gouge a foreign body from your eye. If your eye is smarting for one reason or another you may try boric acid washes or Collyrium solution. The eye is a dangerous area to treat by yourself unless you know exactly what the cause of the problem is.

Fainting

The most common cause of fainting is simply emotional shock. You should have something on hand to treat fainting. Spirits of ammonia does very well, and you can get either the ampoules that you crack, or a solution of spirits of ammonia, which you pour into a teaspoon and hold under the person's nose. If the person continues to be unconscious, then you should consult your physician.

Fever

Since there are many viral illnesses about the community to which all of us are susceptible at times, I see no reason why a layman can't take care of an acute fever, at least until he can consult his doctor to find out what the exact cause is. Aspirin is the mainstay of treatment for acute fever, and you may take as many as three aspirin every four hours if you are an adult. Children should take only one grain every four hours for each year of age up to five years, and then they can take five grains or one adult aspirin every four hours. In addition to aspirin you can give alcohol sponges to your child or yourself when you have fever. The best way to do this is to pour a half bottle of ethyl alcohol into a tub about three or four inches full and lie in the water. The water should be lukewarm. The temperature will come down pretty rapidly under these circumstances. For a child you may want to take turkish towels and dip them in this bath water solution and then put them around the child. This is where a rubber sheet comes in handy, so that you can apply the sponges without dampening the bed.

Hangover

Anyone who has consumed excessive amounts of alcohol on a periodic basis knows what a hangover is. With a hangover you may have nausea and vomiting or gastrointestinal symptoms, or you may have a severe headache. For the nausea and vomiting I think an antacid, such as Maalox, milk of magnesia or Gelusil, is extremely helpful, but your physician could prescribe Compazine suppositories or Tigan suppositories, which would help even more. For the headache there are two drugs that seem to be extremely effective over all the others that you can use. This is a combination of aspirin and one of the amphetamines, dexedrine. One to two taken every four hours is very effective. You must have a prescription from your doctor for this, however. If you do not wish to go to your doctor you may use aspirin, but you should take it with milk. Tomato juice seems to be an excellent drink to start the morning off with. Of course, some people cure their hangovers with another shot of whiskey or another beer, but this is not advisable.

Headaches and other pain

Aspirin is the mainstay for treatment of headaches and, as I said before, in the treatment of fever, you can give as many as three aspirin every four hours for adults with a headache. It has not been shown that combinations of aspirin with caffeine and phenacetin are any more effective than aspirin alone. Your doctor can prescribe for you a more potent analgesic for both pain and headache in the form of Darvon,

Ponstel or Talwin. It is unnecessary for him to give you a narcotic such as codeine except in extreme cases. In any case, it would not be wise to keep a narcotic on hand for fear that the children may get it.

Hemorrhoids

Once you have been diagnosed as having hemorrhoids, you will continue to have problems with them intermittently for the rest of your life unless you have surgery. It is wise for you to keep something on hand to combat the ill effects. People with hemorrhoids may have occasional rectal bleeding at the time of their problems, and this is not a serious thing. If you have pain with your hemorrhoids there is no reason why you cannot treat yourself, at least in the beginning. Of course, if it persists then you should consult your physician. One method of treating painful hemorrhoids is with Preparation H. Wyanoid suppositories may be obtained from your physician, and these are a soothing suppository for treatment of hemorrhoids. Warm sitz baths in a tub with maybe two to three inches of water and three to four teaspoons of salt often help, and these should be done at least twice a day. You should make sure that your stools are soft while you are treating hemorrhoids, and to do this you should have a lot of bulk in your diet or take a tablespoon or two of mineral oil each night.

Insomnia

Most Americans suffer from loss of sleep on one night or another during the month, and it is normal to miss a night's sleep once a month or less. You can get almost as much rest by just lying awake in bed relaxing as you can by being totally asleep, so I wouldn't worry about missing an occasional night's sleep. If you find yourself getting nervous about it, get up and read or do something else, such as a hobby. People who have chronic difficulty sleeping, of course, should consult their physician. But if you have a big day ahead of you and you need to get a good night's sleep, it is well to have something on hand to take. Your doctor can give you a prescription for chloral hydrate, a pretty harmless drug. He may also prescribe either Placidyl, Dalmane, or Doriden. A teaspoon of elixir of phenobarbital might serve the same purpose.

Lacerations

Lacerations all the way through the skin, more than a quarter of an inch wide must be sutured, and therefore you must take the victim—usually a child—to the emergency room. Superficial lacerations, that is, the ones that don't go all through the skin, are usually treated by a layman. It is wise to have two-by-four gauze as well as one- to two-inch size bandage and one-half to one-inch adhesive tape available for this. I do not recommend applying iodine or merthiolate to these wounds. It is much better to just wash them off with soap or Phisohex and apply a dressing if the bleeding continues. If there is dirt in the wound then you must have this removed with forceps. If you cannot do it then let your doctor do it. If you haven't had tetanus toxoid for more than four years and the wound appears dirty, then you must get a tetanus shot.

Superficial burns and abrasions

First or second degree burns and abrasions may be simply scrubbed with Phisohex or a good soap and left open in most cases. This is where Vaseline has been erroneously used. I abhor the use of Vaseline because it only macerates the skin first and contributes to infection. Merthiolate and iodine are poisonous to the skin and therefore only burn the skin further under these circumstances. You want a good crust to form over the burn or abrasion; gentian violet, one to two percent, may be more valuable for this than any of the above. I am sure your doctor would be happy to give you a prescription for this to have on hand. If you simply wash the burn or abrasion and keep it open this is just as effective.

Vaginal irritation

There are a lot of women who treat vaginal itches and vaginal discharges themselves. I'm against this. However, there is nothing wrong with a woman douching herself once or twice a month following the menstrual cycle. The vinegar douches or Massengill douche are very excellent, but a persistent itch or persistent vaginal discharge should be checked by a doctor.

Summary

To summarize, it is permissible for people to treat themselves for the above illnesses as long as they consult a physician should these conditions persist.

PERIODS OF LIFE

Breast-Feeding

I strongly recommend breast-feeding to all mothers. There are many reasons that I recommend breast-feeding. First of all, it has recently been discovered that there are antibodies in the mother's breast that provide the infant with immunity against many illnesses. In addition, breast-feeding gives a tremendous amount of security to the infant and has a tremendous psychological value for the child. Furthermore, breast milk is always warm to the proper temperature and is always available day and night, without the waste of time to prepare formula. And, finally, breast milk comes in a nice package. There are benefits to the mother, which are often overlooked. The uterus is shrunk to its normal size more rapidly, so that there is less likelihood of post partum bleeding. The psychological value to the mother is also great. In some cases breast-feeding does have contraceptive value.

Is it dangerous?

Breast-feeding is not dangerous. The only possible danger is if the breasts crack from the baby's sucking too hard and infection develops. However, if the mother keeps the breasts oiled with cocoa butter or similar substance, this will rarely occur. Contrary to popular belief, the breasts do not get saggy and ugly-looking from breast feeding. Breast-feeding may have to be discontinued should the mother develop an acute illness. If the mother has a chronic illness, such as tuberculosis, which is contagious, breast-feeding must be discouraged. If the mother is taking medication at any time she may not need to discontinue breast feeding, because it will not invariably pass over into the milk. It is extremely desirable for the mother to breast-feed her baby; however, no mother should be forced to breast-feed. If she definitely has an antagonism toward it, it is wise for her to use a formula instead.

Death

What is death?

Death is the absence or cessation of life. It used to be that death could not be pronounced until the heart stopped spontaneously. Now death can be pronounced if the brain has ceased to function and life in the other parts of the body cannot be maintained without mechanical assistance. In this way many organs can be used for transplants.

How can I accept it?

Dying is really nothing to be afraid of. I have seen very few patients get frightened during the last hours of life, when they know there is no hope. Of course, those who believe in God and an afterlife usually accept the final truth best of all. I don't like to tell people they have cancer or some other incurable disease, but I will not lie if they ask. I'm surprised how well the majority accept it. If our churches are doing their job, we should be well prepared to accept death. Death is part of life. We must die so that someone else can take our place. If we love our children then we can be happier about dying, because we know that we are leaving a vacancy for them to fill. Life is in an intricate balance and we would become overpopulated and all starve if some of us didn't die when others are born. Is there an afterlife? I believe there is, if not in another world then right here on earth in our children and in our children's children.

Do you believe in mercy killing?

If mercy killing means administering a drug to someone to hasten death when death is inevitable, then I am against it. To do that is tantamount to murder. However, it is no crime to stop drugs or other medical treatment when they are only prolonging dying instead of life. The question is: Are we to prolong life for a few days at the expense of a great deal of suffering by the patient and the family? I recall a patient with an inoperable brain tumor, who was in a coma for several months. His family visited the hospital daily at great expense and grief. Had his intravenous feedings been stopped sooner a lot of this could have been avoided. Recently, I resuscitated a patient in cardiac arrest. Life returned to his heart but not to his brain. He could not breathe without a mechanical respirator. After discussion with the family the respirator was stopped. Naturally he was pronounced dead a few moments later. Some patients will cry, "You are playing God!" My answer to that is that physicians decided to play God when, with public sanction by licensing, they undertook to prolong life by interfering with the natural course of a disease. In my opinion, it is no crime to choose not to interfere at certain times. The family should be aware of this choice in advance so that they have the option of calling another physician in to take over the case if they do not agree.

AUTOPSY

What is involved in an autopsy?

Most autopsies could be as simple as an exploratory operation during life. In large medical centers pathologists may remove sections of each organ for teaching and research purposes, but the organs are nevertheless put back in place. The family should request a limited autopsy when they feel so inclined, and not just refuse it altogether.

Why have an autopsy?

You should request an autopsy so that you can find out if your parents or relatives have a hereditary disease that you may get later in life. For example, if you found that your father had severe hardening of the arteries at an early age you could take measures to prevent it. Beyond this an autopsy advances medical science immensely. Many people donate thousands of dollars to research but refuse an autopsy, which is worth much more. Tissue sections can be used for research in the disease the patient had. The value of various drugs used during treatment can be better assessed. Your doctor can learn by his mistakes, if there were any.

Marriage

Most people marry today because they love each other. It used to be that people frequently married for money, social position, to please their parents, or because of pregnancy. Not any more. However, is love the main ingredient of a happy marriage? What holds a marriage together? I recently asked a group of three hundred people I was lecturing what holds their marriages together. You'd be surprised what I came up with.

Love

Actually, only a quarter of the people I asked felt love was the most important thing holding their marriage together. Yet most of them felt they married for love. I suspect the discrepancy exists because the initial infatuation has worn off for most married couples. The initial infatuation is really love, but it is physical and emotional love. It is love of another person's body and personality, and I believe it wears off partly because it is not embellished with a love of the other person's mind and soul. Intellectual and spiritual incompatibilities become more significant once people have settled down to the everyday business of living together. For two people to be happily married and develop their love, they must be compatible sexually, emotionally, intellectually, spiritually, and socially. The Lord said, "Love me with all your heart, mind, and soul," and I believe we like the same love.

Sexual compatibility

Fortunately, today with the birth control pill some couples find out whether they are sexually compatible before marriage. I believe premarital relations are permissible under one circumstance: when a couple is engaged and both are certain they would marry the other if circumstances (such as pregnancy) forced it. At least this would prevent people who are sexually incompatible from tying the knot.

Actually, very few couples will be perfectly compatible sexually. This is so because men desire sex daily, particularly when they are first married, and women only weekly or even less. This is understandable physiologically, in view of the fact that women lay only one egg a month, while men are laying "eggs" (sperm) daily. Yet a woman can enjoy sex daily if the husband knows the right techniques to stimulate her (see *All You Wanted to Know About Sex But Were Afraid to Ask,* by Dr. David Reuben). Many arguments in the first months of marriage are on this issue. The young wife thinks her husband is oversexed because he wants it everyday, and the new husband feels his wife doesn't really love him because she refuses him so often.

Women also menstruate once a month. It's perfectly all right to have relations during this time, but most couples don't know this and many husbands won't anyway. During her period a woman may be nasty and depressed. Her husband may become unnecessarily introspective or react hostilely unless he understands this.

Another period of sexual incompatibility is pregnancy. The husband is told to abstain during the last months and for a few weeks after delivery. Finally, many women become depressed and sometimes frigid during menopause. Men must understand these differences between their physiology and that of their wives if the marriage is to survive and, more important, if their love is to survive.

Emotional compatibility

This involves the sensitivity to each other's needs. This is a sixth sense and just comes naturally if you really love someone. When you're in love there is a little voice inside you that's always telling you something you can do to please your lover. It also tells you when he or she is hurt or in distress. You should be able to read each other's mind. Helping your loved one out is no effort, and you don't expect anything in return. Some people are just plain less sensitive to the emotional or physical needs of others. Yet even these people respond remarkably when they are in love. This emotional compatibility involves remembering birthdays and anniversaries. It involves telling each other not only that you love each other but that "you're great." You must build each other's ego. This is genuine when you're in love, but even if you're not it will help your marriage.

Intellectual compatibility

Your marriage is more likely to be a success if you marry someone with about your I.Q. and your level of education.

I think it is nice if the man is a little bit smarter, but even if he isn't, his wife should make him think he is. This is one way to boost his ego, just as he should tell her how beautiful she is. A college graduate shouldn't marry a factory worker.

A doctor might be very unhappy married to a woman lawyer because he could not feel the slight intellectual superiority he needs. Some people have another term for intellectual compatibility; it is *communication.* A couple who can't communiate on the same level will be very unhappy or bored with each other. But communication involves not only intellectual compatibility but also emotional compatibility and love. You must be motivated to fulfill the other person's needs.

Spiritual compatibility

I can't imagine being happily married to an atheist any more than they would probably be happy with me. Yet we might have a lot to talk about if we could control our emotions. Today more and more people, including Catholics and Jews, are marrying outside their faith. The difficulties of "mixed" marriages seem to rise out of how the children will be raised. In my opinion, this should be settled before the marriage, but the child should be given his own choice by the time he is eight years old. Spiritual compatibility involves not only going to the same church. It involves appreciating the same aesthetic beauty (the sky, trees, etc.), music, animals, and poetry. It involves interest in the same sports. Of course, these could be grouped under social compatibility also.

Social compatibility

It is most wise for a couple contemplating marriage to be socially compatible. This means they should be from the same class of people, race and nationality. They should like the same hobbies—music, sports, theater, etc. Many wives who love dancing often complain to me that their husbands can't dance. On the other hand, the cheerleader who falls for the high school football hero may find they have very little else in common, and what you have in common matters a great deal.

The law

A lot of marriages are held together by a legal piece of paper. Once a couple have accumulated a lot of assets they are afraid to part with them. Women may become especially attached to the house and furniture. A husband doesn't like splitting a large income with a wife he no longer loves. So they stay together, grin and bear it. A long divorce proceeding is trying and embarrassing to most people. Many are afraid of what their parents, neighbors, and other members of society will think. Even though as many as fifty percent of marriages in one state end in divorce, divorced people don't feel they are accepted.

The legal problems could be settled before marriage. If we entered marriage with a partnership agreement including a dissolution clause like all other business partnerships have, then the fear of divorce proceedings and what will happen to our material possessions could be eliminated. With a divorce agreement worked out in advance, love might be turned to more often to keep the marriage together. It would be a marriage based on love and compatibility. Judges should refuse to marry people unless they have had several hours of instruction in marriage along these lines.

Religion

I am sure that many marriages are held together because of the fear of God. The Catholic church makes it clear that they are against divorce by excommunication, and while other churches may not make a penalty they are nevertheless strongly against it. It is perfectly sound for the churches to be against it, since the family is sacred to religion; but I am sure God would forgive the divorced, and we should do likewise. If the church were permissive in this regard couples might divorce without much thought. Yet the church has a responsibility to prepare people better for marriage. Religious leaders should refuse to perform the wedding ceremony without several hours of instruction in marriage.

Children

Of all the bonds holding marriages together, children are probably the most important. The majority of the three hundred people I asked put children first. This is as it should be. Children need two parents, not just one. Many children involved in crime come from broken homes. Many children who need psychiatric help come from broken homes. A child needs a mother's love and a father's discipline. Actually he should get both from each parent. However, it is rare for one parent to be able to supply both in adequate amounts to raise a well-adjusted child. Many couples think twice about a divorce because they are afraid of the psychological effects on their children. If the children are all over twelve years of age these effects can be minimal. They can be kept at a minimum if both parents continue to show love to the children and are allowed to. Parents who use the children as pawns in their battle with each other are committing a cardinal sin. They should never talk down to or degrade one another in front of the children.

How to settle arguments

Couples who love one another and are compatible in most respects have little difficulty in settling arguments. Yet disagreements occur from time to time. Sensible objective discussion will often settle the issue if emotional overtones can be kept down. A common impediment to a settlement is that one or the other party may bring up mistakes the other has made in the past as part of his persuasive technique. This is to be condemned. I call it heavy artillery. For example, the wife may remind the husband about the time he went out with a broad in Chicago when she is trying to convince him she needs a new living room suite.

Who is going to have the final say in case of a tie or stalemate? I think that since women are well educated today and many of them consider themselves equal to men the final decision should be divided between the two members. The final decision regarding what kind of carpeting or furniture should be in the home, what kind of clothes should be purchased for the children, etc., should lie in the hands of the wife, as long as her needs are not extravagant and not above the income of the family. The decision of what foods should be put on the table should be in her hands. However, the wise wife will consult her husband on these matters so that she can get his opinion before she finally makes up her mind. On the other hand, the decision as to where the husband works and what kind of work he does, how many hours he works, and how he gets to work should be largely his. Here, again, he would be wise to consult his wife before making a final decision. Decisions regarding the management of the children should be a joint proposition, although if the wife is home most of the day she will take this responsibility more often than the husband and bother him only when things get out of control. When the two are home together they must face the children jointly, and whatever one says the other should back up. There should be no disagreement in front of the children. A disagreement should be discussed in private.

There are undoubtedly modifications of the above recommendations that must be applied when both the wife and husband work, and there must be some changes when neither of the two work. If both the husband and wife work, then the responsibilities of the home, kids, cooking meals, and ironing clothes, etc., may be shared by both members. However, this produces many problems, which I will not go into at this time. When neither works the husband will often pitch in and share the responsibility of the home because of sheer boredom. He may well get on his wife's nerves, and this will create disharmony between the two members.

Freedom in marriage

This is another problem that can break up a happy home. What does each member of the marriage do with his or her free time, and who has the right to decide what he or she *should* do with this free time? How many nights should the husband be allowed to stay out each week? How often should the wife be allowed to go out, either alone or with her husband? What obligations should each member of the marriage have to each other in this area? I can answer very succinctly by saying neither party should be obligated to the other for one minute of his or her free time. The decision about what they do with their free time should be entirely their own. Obviously, if the two are in love the majority of the free time will be spent together. But when one party in the marriage decides that the other is obligated to spend all his or her free time with the first, trouble starts.

Assuming that there are no children and that the husband provides a good living, he should be entitled to spend as much time outside of the home as he desires. His free time should be his own. Likewise, if the wife is doing an adequate job of housekeeping she should be able to spend as much time outside of the home as she wants. If she wants to take a vacation she must provide a suitable substitute for taking care of the job of housekeeping. What I am recommending is that husbands and wives stop insisting that the other is obligated to spend all their free time together.

If there are children in the marriage, then obviously the husband should spend more free time at home. How much time the father should spend with the children will vary with the marriage. It certainly varies with the children's age. When the children are very young they are more in need of the mother rather than the father. As they mature they will want him to spend more time with them, but when they get into their teens they hardly care if he is around. Yet he should be around for disciplinary problems. If the wife spends much of her working hours at home, doing housekeeping chores, she is exposed to the children during the day, and therefore in the evening it is not as important for her to be around, particularly when the children are older. This is why many wives can work after the children reach school age and it doesn't affect the personality or development of the children in any way whatsoever. I feel that to force each other to spend every moment at home is nonsense. This is not to say that marriages where the two members are very happy doing everything—and I mean everything—together do not exist, but in this type of relationship I'm sure there is rarely any feeling of obligation between one another. In other words, they are not being forced to stay together every minute of the day. In those circumstances involving obligation one or the other will most certainly rebel. On the other hand, there are marriages in which the two are very happy doing everything separately, and here again I'm sure the decision to do everything separately was made freely and independently. The marriage could not otherwise be happy.

In summary, no marriage is perfect. It is necessary for each partner to compromise on many occasions. With love strengthened and renewed by compatibility this will be easy in most cases. If we weigh the advantages of our marriages against the disadvantages of being single and divorced we will usually conclude that marriage is a good institution.

Menopause

What is the menopause?

Menopause is the gradual dwindling of the amount of bleeding at the time of your period and the gradual increase in the amount of time between your periods. Periods become irregular and eventually they cease. Actually, the fact that they cease is the main symptom of menopause. Some physiological changes of menopause may begin as early as twenty-nine years of age and there are some authorities that feel it may begin at twenty-six years in a few women. Therefore there is a wide variability of the onset of menopause. Some women begin menopause in their fifties. The mean age of menopause is forty-four years of age.

What causes the menopause?

The ovaries, which are the woman's reproductive glands, during their entire reproductive life produce several eggs, but there is a limit to the number of eggs that they produce. The lining of the eggs, or if you want to consider it the "egg shells," contain tiny cells that secrete hormones. The number of eggs produced by the ovaries declines in number as one approaches the age of menopause. With fewer cells from the lining of these eggs producing hormones, the amount of female hormones gradually dwindles. However, most ovaries do secrete a small amount of hormones throughout the life of the woman, but after menopause this is not enough to stimulate the growth of the lining of the womb. Thus the periodic sloughing of the lining of the uterus with the associated bleeding ceases! After the menopause the adrenal gland takes over in the secretion of some estrogen hormones. Therefore, not all women suffer a tremendous reduction of the amount of estrogen in their blood.

What are the symptoms and signs of menopause?

The signs vary from one patient to another. I have patients complaining of depression, fatigue, or insomnia, which are more indefinite symptoms and can be related to their emotional make-up. Then I have others who complain of hot flashes or flushes, which are so typical of menopause. The hot flushes are a burning and reddening of the face and upper chest. This is sometimes just a cold chill running up the spine. It may begin at the feet and go to the head or start from the abdomen and go to the head. In any case it is a periodic phenomenon lasting maybe one to five minutes, rarely more than ten minutes. Some women have two to three of these a day and others have ten to fifteen a day. This is about the only symptom that can be definitely ascribed to the menopause other than the fact that one ceases having periods.

Irregular bleeding, of course, is another symptom of menopause. Sometimes there is an increase in bleeding, because the growth in the lining of the uterus is irregular and polypoid masses can form. On the other hand, some of the heavy bleeding may be related to the development of tumors, such as fibroids, endometrial (the lining of the womb) or cervical cancer, so this is a time of life when a woman must have frequent checks by her physician for the possibility of cancer. In the vast majority these examinations turn out negative, so there is no cause for alarm just because a person is having irregular or excessive bleeding. Some women have tension headaches or develop migraine headaches at the time of menopause. This is another symptom. Menopausal depression can be severe (an involutional melancholia), but very few women require institutionalization for psychiatric treatment, contrary to popular belief. A few women have a loss of libido (sexual desire) but for others there is an increase. Perhaps this is partly due to the fact that women no longer have a fear of pregnancy and also don't have to worry about periods and the messiness involved with this. Perhaps the worst symptoms are not the hot flushes but the depression, insomnia, and loss of appetite. Some authorities do not believe that the estrogen has anything to do with such symptoms but that most of these symptoms are psychological. These clinicians feel that some women at the time of menopause have a "castration complex" because they are losing their reproductive capacity and can no longer fulfill their purpose in life (having children). Some feel they should end their lives. The menopause also comes at an age when these mothers are experiencing their children leaving the nest. They must become involved in something else, such as a job or a new responsibility in the community, if they are to avoid depression.

What can I do about the menopause?

Up until the last ten to fifteen years the only treatment was psychiatric care, and as I mentioned a lot of these women were hospitalized for psychiatric care. Some of them began analysis that probably should have begun years ago in their lives, but because of the tremendous blow to their physiology from the menopause they finally get to a psychiatrist. But for the vast majority of women there is no need for psychiatric help.

When they begin the symptoms of depression, insomnia, and hot flushes, etc., they need *hormone replacement,* mainly replacement of *estrogen* hormones. This need may develop as early as twenty-nine, as I have mentioned above. I have several women in my practice that require this at the age of thirty-five or thirty-six, when they are still having regular periods and the amount of blood passed during their periods has not diminished significantly. For the women who are still having periods we must give the estrogen periodically in very low doses. However, those women who have stopped their periods can often receive low doses steadily without producing any severe complications. Other women do require periodic doses and may return to having periods regularly. Many patients require tranquilizers and sedatives to get through the night, but I find this is only needed temporarily until the body has responded to oral hormone therapy. To get some of the women started I find it is very valuable to give them a shot of estrogen hormone. Each physician will choose his own method of giving estrogen, and this will be the one he has had the best results with. Again, the dosage and the frequency of replacement therapy varies with the individual.

Is hormone therapy dangerous?

There is no danger in giving estrogen. The greatest fear of prescribing estrogen therapy ten years ago was cancer. This fear has been found to be fallacious. In fact, fewer women taking estrogen have cancer than those who have not. Breast cancer is the only one that may have some increased incidence in people who have a family history of breast cancer. The only other problem with estrogen replacement therapy is the fact that sometimes women have recurrence of their menstrual cycles and they do not like the messy bleeding. There may be excessive menstrual bleeding or breakthrough bleeding. This is no problem; the estrogen can be withdrawn for a short time and normal functioning reestablished. Some women have required a D and C but these are few.

Is the menopause dangerous?

The menopause is dangerous in the few cases where a woman becomes so depressed she commits suicide! Very few women really go off their "rocker," and most of them could pass through this without estrogen therapy but now that we have this marvelous drug it seems ridiculous to withhold it and make a woman suffer through the two to five years when she has emotional instability and hot flushes.

How long must I continue the therapy?

This will vary with the individual, but many of these women require replacement therapy for the rest of their lives. I'm amazed that physicians have little qualms about giving thyroid replacement for the rest of a person's life after they have established a diagnosis of hypothyroidism (underactive thyroid), but with estrogens they seem to feel that this should only be used for a short time. Since this is a natural substance, there is no reason why it cannot be continued indefinitely. Your adrenal gland may take over the secretion of estrogen hormone, but this is not likely to be sufficient for your needs. You could have repeated urine tests for hormone evaluations and pap smears for hormone evaluations while taking therapy, and if you do not change after discontinuing therapy you may not need to continue indefinitely. However, the best way to decide on how to continue the hormone therapy is by the patient's clinical picture, i.e., symptoms.

What can I do to prevent menopause?

Don't allow your surgeon to take out your ovaries unless absolutely necessary, even though a hysterectomy may be necessary. Other than this there is nothing you can do. Women who take birth control pills for a long period of time can delay menopause for a certain number of years.

Menstruation

What is menstruation?

Menstruation is the onset of cyclic vaginal bleeding, or the beginning of womanhood for females. At this point in her life a woman is physiologically an adult. It is very unfortunate in our society that one reaches physiological adulthood before one can get married and begin having children. Immaturity is to a certain extent imposed on our children. Many things regarding sex, particularly menstruation, are not explained to our children. Therefore, when many young adult women begin having periods they are frightened to death. Fortunately, with the better mass media of communication a lot of this ignorance has been removed. All parents should explain menstruation to their daughters. Menstruation is the physiological bleeding from the womb (uterus) through the vagina, which occurs between twenty and thirty-five days every month. It lasts anywhere from three to ten days in a normal adult. The blood is usually dark and it usually does not clot. The bleeding is often associated with crampy pain in the lower abdomen and in the low back, and a woman will use anywhere from three to six pads a day normally or two to five tampons per day, but this will vary with the individual woman. If the menstrual period lasts beyond ten days or if there is a need for more than eight sanitary pads per day a physician should be consulted about the problem.

What causes menstruation?

A woman lays about three hundred forty to three hundred sixty eggs during her adult life and she lays about one a month. Each month the lining of the womb is prepared to receive the egg "hoping" that it will be fertilized by a male sperm. If the egg does not become fertilized and therefore does not implant into the lining of the womb, then the lining is sloughed off and passes through the vagina along with the egg and some blood. What causes this lining of the womb to develop?

There is a shell around the egg as it is growing in the ovary, the place where all the eggs are produced. This shell produces hormones of two different types, which help prepare the lining of the womb. One of the hormones is estrogen. This is produced early in the growth of the egg in the ovary, and it produces an increased number of cells in the lining of the womb. About the middle of the cycle a second hormone, progesterone, is manufactured by the ovary, and this produces a secretory lining of the womb. After the middle of the month both estrogen and progesterone are being secreted by the ovary.

About the middle of the month the egg is released and it is passed from the ovary through the fallopian tubes into the womb, where it may have the opportunity to meet a male sperm and therefore become fertilized. If it becomes fertilized then it digs into the lining of the womb and begins to grow. Eventually the placenta of the developing embryo produces chorionic gonadotropin, a hormone which stimulates further secretion of progesterone and estrogen by the ovary. If the egg is not fertilized then it passes out through the womb and is in a sense laid. However, one cannot see the egg because it is too small. Because the womb did not receive a fertilized egg its lining is sloughed off within twenty to thirty-five days. The slough is passed mainly in the form of blood and small particles of endometrial lining.

Menstruation may begin anywhere from ten years of age to eighteen or nineteen years of age. I have been consulted frequently by mothers who were concerned about their daughters' not having their periods before they were sixteen. I feel it is foolish to worry about a complete endocrine diagnostic work-up until after the daughter has reached sixteen years of age. Then hormone assays on the urine and various other procedures can be done, as well as checking into the thyroid metabolism, pituitary metabolism, etc. Menstruation usually stops between forty-five and fifty-five years of age. This is because the woman stops laying eggs. At this time, as we have discussed in the chapter on menopause, a woman may require replacement of hormones. Therefore it may be possible to continue menstruation until a woman is sixty-five or seventy, depending on how long she takes the hormones and if she takes the hormones in a cyclical fashion. Patients who take hormones under these circumstances should not be alarmed by having their periods continue.

During the menstruation some women douche every day. I think this is foolish. I think a woman should refrain from douching until the end of the cycle, and then this should be the only douche she performs during the entire month. As mentioned above some women douche after intercourse and regularly two or three times a week, whether they have intercourse or not. This practice should be stopped.

There are a lot of old wives' tales about menstruation. It has been called the "curse" for women. This should not be. Puberty should be a delightful time in a woman's life, a time when she can call herself a woman. She should have a tremendous uplift in her ego because now she can perform the most important function that she was created for; that is, to have children. Also, I would caution young adults and their mothers about the seriousness of a great deal of bleeding. This is rarely anything serious. Even though the amount of blood may appear great, it is very unusual for a person to lose more than a half a pint of blood during a menstrual cycle. If the young adult woman has an adequate diet she will probably get enough iron, but it is not unusual for girls in their teens to eat poorly, because they are running from one place to another and they eat a lot of cafeteria food. Therefore I advise taking an iron supplement to make up for the blood lost during each cycle.

A lot of parents ask whether tampons are preferred over sanitary pads. In general, this is a matter of personal preference. Sometimes fungus or bacterial infections are introduced into the vagina using the tampons; therefore the menstrual pads are probably safer physiologically. On the other hand, menstrual pads lead to a particular odor coming from women, and sometimes they are annoying in between the legs, so it is understandable that they are objectionable to many women. What did women do before they had these two items to protect them? I do not know. I would imagine they bathed frequently or wore a certain type of cloth to protect themselves. In this sense menstruation is certainly a "curse" because it requires a woman to wear apparel that otherwise would be unnecessary. The bleeding cannot be controlled like urination and therefore can be very embarrassing at times. Why God did not make women a little more able to control this I do not know. There is however a muscle around the vagina that if controlled properly should be able to make a woman continent of her menstrual bleeding so that she could release it whenever she desired to. Perhaps the use of Kotex and Tampax has made this muscle lazy. The incontinence of vaginal bleeding may be the result of man's own ignorance.

In the discussion of menstruation one cannot exclude *premenstrual tension* and *cramps.* Premenstrual tension is a very common condition in young adult females before they have had any children, but for some it can continue into the thirties and early forties. This is a complex of symptoms, including depression, puffiness of the breasts, swelling of the eyes, and swelling of other parts of the body including the hands and legs, that usually occurs within five to ten days prior to the onset of bleeding. It may be associated with back pain, lower abdominal pain, and cramps. This condition is probably due to increased fluid in the body caused by the progesterone at this time of the cycle. It is probably a bit more common in the neurotic or anxious woman but it occurs in many normal women also. The best way to treat this condition is to take a diuretic (page 66), in other words, a water pill, which releases a lot of the fluid, makes the breasts more supple and in many cases relieves the depression.

Menstrual cramps are a natural reaction of the womb to the slough material that is coming through the cervix. The womb must expel this material, and sometimes in women who have had no children it must expel this through a very small opening in the cervix. In these women delivery of the blood and sloughed epithelium from the endometrium is similar to delivering or expelling a baby. The cramps, however, do not usually occur at five- or ten-minute intervals and may increase to one- to two-minute intervals because, of course, periodically some of the material is expelled. Cramps are not a dangerous thing or a sign that a woman has cancer.

There are three major causes of severe menstrual cramps. One is a very small opening of the cervix. This can be relieved by dilation of the cervix. Some women who have this problem are relieved of their menstrual cramps immediately after having their first child. So, for some women who have menstrual cramps my advice is get married and have children! The second cause of menstrual cramps is simple retention of fluid in the walls of the womb itself, making the cervix very puffy and the whole womb very puffy. This can be relieved by a diuretic. The third cause of menstrual cramps is psychological. A lot of women with emotional problems in their family or difficulties with their husbands complain more bitterly of "normal" cramps, which become a defense against the husband or a way of getting sympathy, etc. The treatment of this condition is discussion of the problem with your physician or psychiatrist. Sometimes deep psychoanalysis is required.

A fourth cause of menstrual cramps is actual pathology, in other words disease of the womb. A retroverted uterus is a common cause. The womb is tipped backward so that it is more difficult for the uterine musculature to contract and expel the blood. In addition, a fibroid tumor, polyps, or cancer of the womb may cause menstrual cramps. The doctor will certainly be able to determine whether you have one of the diseases mentioned. Diseases of the womb are probably the least common cause of menstrual cramps. It is therefore very unlikely that anything serious will happen to you if you do not consult your doctor about menstrual cramps.

Old Age

I have had many patients tell me that other doctors frequently ascribe their condition to "old age." In my opinion no disease is due to old age! Old age as a diagnosis is really a substitute for our ignorance. If I were to approach every elderly patient's problem with the idea that it was probably due to old age, I would have missed many diagnoses of conditions that are easily treated. For example, at sixty-seven years old a lawyer had been told for the past four years that his fatigue and depression were due to old age. Yet, diagnostic studies proved he had an underactive parathyroid gland. After proper treatment he was able to return to an active law practice at the age of sixty-eight.

Hardening of the arteries, or arteriosclerosis, is not due to old age. Senility is probably not due to old age either. We will eventually find that in this condition there is merely a premature deficiency of a certain enzyme in the nerve tissue.

Some scientists have developed a theory that there is a biological time clock for humans and their individual tissues. Yet we are able to keep tissues alive for years beyond their regular life span in the proper culture medium. This certainly shoots holes in that theory. Certainly there is wear and tear on certain structures because of long and continued use, but this is not the same as "old age." For example, many older people have osteoarthritis of the knee and ankle joints. Yet young football players get the same type of arthritis from hard and continued use. The bone changes of the spine that seem to accompany aging are seen in many people who do heavy labor. I am certain the day will come when "old" will be replaced by the word "worn." When we refer to human beings who have lived the longest we will be thinking in numbers only and not in terms of approaching death. Science will discover a way to keep us living indefinitely. Then we will all be faced with the moral problem of deciding when we should die.

Pregnancy

It is unnecessary to define pregnancy, nor is it necessary to discuss the cause. One wonders how long it took primitive man to learn the cause, since there are nine months between conception and birth. It takes intercourse at a certain time of the month to cause conception. Also, the period of gestation (development of the child in the womb) may vary a great deal.

What are the symptoms and signs of pregnancy?

Most women realize they are pregnant when they miss a period. There are many other indications. The breasts become swollen and tender. There is nausea and vomiting, particularly in the early morning. There is frequency of urination and a copious white discharge. There is bloating and fluid retention and later significant gain of weight. A few women do not realize they are pregnant until their belly bulges or they actually feel life in the fetus (unborn child). On examination the womb is found to be enlarged and the mouth (cervix) and neck (isthmus) are soft as early as the sixth week. The whole womb becomes soft by the twelfth week. The mouth of the womb may be bluish red. A urine test for pregnancy is almost always positive by the fourth week, but it should be repeated when in doubt. Your doctor can also give you pills that will bring on your period if you are not pregnant. This will help establish the diagnosis early. Don't laugh if he has difficulty deciding whether you are or not during the first three months because it isn't always that easy.

What can I do about it?

If you think you are pregnant you should see your doctor as early as possible to establish the diagnosis. Your care is divided into three phases: prenatal (the period before delivery), perinatal (the period of delivery), and postpartum (the period after the delivery).

Prenatal care

You should see your doctor regularly at least once a month from the time you are three months pregnant until you deliver. Your doctor will examine you to be sure you have an adequate birth canal. Otherwise he will plan a Caesarian section. He will check your weight, urine and blood pressure. A rapid increase in weight or blood pressure or the appearance of albumin in the urine may mean that you are getting *toxemia* of pregnancy. In this disease there is spasm of the small arteries all over the body causing hypertension and there is damage to the kidneys causing fluid retention. No one knows the exact cause, but if you restrict your weight gain to twenty-five pounds or less during pregnancy you will go a long way toward preventing it.

On your first visit your doctor will also check your blood type to be sure you are not subject to "RH" babies and your serology to be sure that venereal disease is not passed on to your child. "RH" babies occur when an Rh negative mother conceives with an Rh positive father. The baby's blood is often but not always Rh positive. The mother may form antibodies to the baby's blood and these antibodies cross over into the baby and destroy his blood. This makes him anemic and jaundiced. The condition is known as erythroblastosis fetalis, or "jaundice of the newborn." With proper prenatal care it can be prevented. Your doctor will also check your blood count on your first visit. Iron deficiency and other types of anemia often occur in pregnancy because mothers fail to eat a well-balanced diet. That is why your doctor will usually prescribe a vitamin with iron.

There are many other reasons why you should be checked frequently during pregnancy. You may have twins or triplets and the earlier your doctor knows that the better. He will want to listen for the baby's heart so that he can tell if it is in any distress or not. If he doesn't hear the heart by the end of the sixth month then the baby may be dead or you may have some other condition. X-rays will help in difficult decisions. He must be sure the head is getting into the proper position for delivery. Unusual positions of the baby in the mother may be an indication for a Caesarian section.

Perinatal care

When you begin getting pains in your lower abdomen or lower back at regular intervals, or you start a bloody vaginal discharge, you are probably in or about to be in labor, and it's time to call the doctor and get to the hospital. Some women rupture their "bag of water" (the sack of fluid around the baby) before labor pains or a bloody show begins. They should call the doctor immediately. When you get to the hospital you will get bathed, have an enema, and be put in a labor room. Your doctor will examine you to see how far you have progressed. He can tell this by the amount the mouth of your womb has opened. When it reaches 8-10 cm. or four to five fingers you are ready to be delivered. The nurse can examine you frequently during labor and report her findings to the doctor, allowing him to get some sleep, especially if your labor is going to be long.

Once you are in the delivery room everything will usually be over in a half hour. The type of anesthesia to be given should have been decided between you and your doctor beforehand. You can have spinal, general or local. In *local anesthesia* Novocain is injected around the rectal and vaginal area, and the pudendal nerves, two important nerves supplying the tissues of the birth canal, are blocked. I personally prefer *spinal anesthesia.* The mother feels very little pain and yet the baby breathes sooner when he comes out because he has had no anesthetic in his blood to sedate him. Women who desire natural childbirth should not be discouraged. However, it seems foolish to suffer in this day and age when you can witness the whole delivery anyway.

After you have received anesthesia, the vaginal and rectal area are thoroughly cleansed and painted with Zephiran (an antiseptic solution). You will be catheterized to be sure your bladder is empty so it won't hinder the passage of the baby. With a few good pushes the baby's head will appear at the opening of the vagina. At this point it may be necessary to cut the skin and tissues just beneath the skin on one corner of the vagina to make it big enough to get the baby through. This is called an *episiotomy.* It can be easily sewed up after the baby is delivered. It may be necessary to apply forceps to get the head out at this point. This is not usually a difficult procedure and rarely causes harm. Once the head is out the shoulders, hips and legs follow easily in rapid sequence.

Then the cord is grabbed, tied and cut. The baby's nose and mouth are suctioned and if he doesn't cry at this point he is spanked. Sometimes a tube may be inserted into the trachea and other procedures can be used to induce breathing. After the cord is cut, the placenta (after birth) will usually come out by itself but the inside of the womb should be checked to be sure all of the placenta is removed. If you had an episiotomy this is sutured and you are ready to leave the delivery room for the recovery room.

Postpartum care

Once in the recovery room your blood pressure and pulse are taken regularly and you are examined for bleeding. Postpartum hemorrhage is still a significant complication, although very few women die of this since we have a good supply of matched blood. During the remainder of your hospital stay your blood pressure will be checked to be sure you don't get postpartum toxemia of pregnancy, and your temperature will be checked to be sure you aren't getting an infection of your womb (puerperal sepsis) or episiotomy. The sutures of the episiotomy do not have to be removed. They will dissolve or fall out by themselves.

Breast-feeding

This is a controversial issue, but most physicians believe that breast milk is best. It is easier to digest, supplies the baby with good immunity for some infections, and best of all comes in a nice package. The psychological value to the infant is also important. A lot of mothers who don't breast-feed turn the responsibility of feeding the baby over to the father or some other member of the family. This interrupts a warm and tender relationship. If you are not going to breast-feed, your doctor will give you pills to dry up your milk during the postpartum period.

You should see your doctor again from three to six weeks after the delivery. This is to make sure the womb is getting small again and that the mouth of your cervix and your episiotomy have healed properly. Other problems can be discussed then. It used to be that sexual relations were forbidden during the last three months of pregnancy and the first six weeks afterwards. I now see no harm in intercourse up to two weeks before delivery, and you may commence again two weeks after delivery if your husband is gentle. This is because we have antibiotics to cure any complication.

Is it dangerous?

Pregnancy is a healthy, normal process for most women. Complications such as hemorrhage, toxemia, and infection, which used to kill one in ten mothers, are rare today. I really believe a lot of frigidity in women, especially married women, can be traced to a fear of the complications of pregnancy. Infant mortality is also much lower than it used to be and is nothing to fear. It should be pointed out that while pregnancy is very safe, the birth control pill has even fewer side effects than pregnancy.

How can I prevent it?

Read the chapter on contraceptives.

Raising Children

The fact that so many children are growing up to be antisocial in today's world means that we are failing in raising our children. Just what are parents doing wrong today that they were doing right before? I think the most important things to inculcate in our children are love, honesty, confidentiality and secrecy, and a respect for law and order.

Love

Our children will return or reflect just about as much love as they receive. If Mom and Dad spend a lot of time with them explaining life and giving them physical, as well as emotional and intellectual love, then they will in turn pass this on to their friends and to everyone else they meet when they become adults. Our love for them is not only manifested by buying them presents or giving them material things; it must also be manifested by emotional and physical contact. Some parents shun hugging their children. This creates a definite deficiency in that child. Some children do not require as much love, physical or emotional, as another child, so you must individualize your approach.

Love is also shown by your concern, not only for their happiness but also for their moral character and their ability to take responsibility. A parent's concern with a child's grades in school is a very good way to show love. A mother's discipline of her child is a good way to show love. Tucking your children in bed at night and teaching them to say their prayers and showing them how to love others through their prayers can be a valuable means of showing love. Your love for your children will also be demonstrated when you settle arguments with their friends, or brothers and sisters, in an amiable fashion. The best way for you to show love is by setting an example.

Honesty

Here, again, the child will reflect the exact amount of honesty that is seen in the parents. If the mother is always doing something behind the father's back, then the child will become a sneaky individual also. And vice-versa, if the father is doing things behind the mother's back this will reflect in the child. Dishonesty should be punished immediately. Also, you should admit when you have been dishonest in front of your children. When your child is dishonest towards his friends you must reprimand him immediately.

Secrecy

This is an extremely important characteristic to inculcate in our children. A child who cannot keep secrets and, more important, an adult who cannot keep secrets will be a failure in anything he attempts to do. In any case he can never be a real close friend to anyone unless he can keep secrets. I think this is one of the most deficient areas in our society today. Some women, particularly, are nothing but gossips in their adult life and have no respect for the privacy of others. This is because they were not told to keep secrets as a child. Rewards should be set up for keeping secrets. I like to test my children by giving them a secret to hold for a week or even a month and then giving them a reward for success at the end of that period; but if you are going to have a child that keeps secrets, then you must not tell on him when you promise to keep a secret. For instance, mothers who invariably report the child's mistakes or accidents or disciplinary infringements to the father when he comes home will only cause that child to have little respect for secrecy.

Respect for law and order

Respect for law and order has deteriorated today because of lack of discipline in our homes. For one thing most parents begin discipline too late. Most children are ready for discipline by eight or ten months of age yet I have seen many parents wait till the child is two or three or even six years of age before they start to say "no" to a child. But a child of eight to ten months will easily understand the command "no." The first time you say "no" he will test you to see if he gets the same response by performing the same act. Then he will be conditioned to understand what "no" means. That is why you must back up the "no" with a slap on the rear when he does not listen to you. Above all you must be consistent. You can't say "no" to a certain act one time and say "yes" or avoid or overlook it next time. Every time you say "no," if you find that the child violates it you must back the command up with force at the right time. If you say "no" and do not back it up with force it will lead to anarchy. Some parents will slap a child before they even say anything. This prevents the child from being conditioned to your voice. Other parents will say "no" ten times and never back it up with force. In this case the command becomes meaningless. Proper disciplining is like conditioning a dog to respond to a bell by salivating, as Pavlov did. In Pavlov's experiment the dog instinctively salivated at the sight of meat. Then Pavlov rang a bell prior to giving the meat. Eventually the dog salivated at the sound of the bell. In the same way your child is conditioned to respond to your commands. At first the only withdrawal is when he is struck on the behind, but if you say "no" just before or two commands before then he will eventually be conditioned to the sound of the word "no."

During the years of raising children I strongly believe in punishment. However, the parent who beats his child unmercifully with a belt defeats the purpose of punishment. I don't think any instrument other than the hand should be used to punish the child; use of the hand alone means parent-to-child contact without a weapon. Parents who withhold punishment with the excuse that the child must express himself are to be condemned. I have heard some parents contend that discipline thwarts initiative and creates an inhibited child. Too much discipline may well do that, but too little leads to a confused and insecure child who lacks purpose and direction in his life. More important, there is a lack of respect for law and order when he gets to be an adult. Just as dangerous is inconsistency in discipline. A child who one time gets a smack for a certain act and next time gets praise will undoubtedly lead a confused existence for the rest of his life. Discipline must be administered with love and understanding. As a child gets older it will be unnecessary to strike him. Suitable punishments will be restricting him from watching television or from going out with his friends, making him wear the same clothes every day, or sitting him on a "naughty" step.

In order for discipline to be effective, a child must respect his parents. When children are small they do this because of the difference in size and power, but as they grow older they look for subtle qualities. For example, if the father or mother holds a respected position in society (such as doctor, lawyer, or judge) he may get more respect. Even more important than this is how much one marital partner respects the other partner. A wife can build a lot of respect for the husband by praising him in front of the children. She can describe how important it is that he provides for the home, the clothing, and the food when he is out working. She can also praise him for the responsible job he holds in society. These things should be repeatedly emphasized. Parents should never countermand each other in front of the children or bicker about the other's decision about the children. This is particularly true when one parent disagrees with the disciplinary action the other has taken. They must have a united front before the children. If the child can play one parent against the other then he will lose respect for both and, more important, lose respect for law and order in society.

Responsibility

Children must also learn responsibility early in life. I feel children should be given jobs as early as three and four years of age, if it's only emptying the wastebaskets. They should be paid for this and adequately. There is a great deal of security derived from carrying out a small job and also a great deal of security gained by earning money from this. As they grow older more responsible jobs can be given to them with more money.

In summary the qualities of love, honesty, and secrecy, as well as respect for law and order, and responsibility can be inculcated in your children best by a consistent united approach by both parents and by setting an example for your children

Index